Dr. Spencer Baron's

SECRETS OF THE GAME:
*What Superstar Athletes Can Teach You about
Health, Peak Performance, and Getting Results!*

"If you're having a rough time keeping up with the kids, or finding yourself hitting the wall when it comes to getting critical things done in your life due to a lack of energy, then you owe it to yourself to read this book.. I've known Dr. Spencer Baron since we were kids, and I can tell you he is the real deal. This guy walks the talk and is the go to guy to all the top performers. If he's in your area, do not miss his special presentation."
Carlos Castellanos
Syndicated Cartoonist
Baldo Comics - Co creator

"Ok please put me on the VIP list for the book signing - I want to be first in line! BTW, just returned from Chicago - Team USA Karate trials for Maccabiah Games 2009. I have been appointed to the coaching staff for the Games and served on the Selection Committee to pick our teams. I would love to use your book to keep our team healthy and strong, so bring it on Doc! I have always endorsed your work!"
Caren Lesser
Attorney
Black belt

It appears some of the world's most gifted athletes have learned how to access a set of universal performance secrets. I believe these principals represent the frontier of performance based medicine.

*Spencer Baron, D.C., D.A.C.B.S.P. has taken his experience in working with elite and professional athletes thru out his career and distilled these "performance principals" into a simple yet comprehensive formula for success, not just in athletics, **but in life**!*
Dr. James L. Holding
Board Certified Chiropractic Sports Physician
National Hockey League - Washington Capitals
Team Chiropractor
www.drholding.com

Dr. Spencer Baron's

SECRETS OF THE GAME:

What Superstar Athletes Can Teach You about Health, Peak Performance, and Getting Results!

Spencer Baron

New York

Secrets of the Game
What Superstar Athletes can Teach you About Health, Peak Performance and Getting Results

ISBN 978-1-60037-617-7

Library of Congress Control Number: 2009924313

Photos for cover by Lucy Unsworth [www.unsworthphotography.com]
Cover design by Rachel Lopez [rachel@r2cdesign.com]

MORGAN · JAMES
THE ENTREPRENEURIAL PUBLISHER

Morgan James Publishing, LLC
1225 Franklin Ave., STE 325
Garden City, NY 11530-1693
Toll Free 800-485-4943
www.MorganJamesPublishing.com

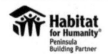

In an effort to support local communities, raise awareness and funds, Morgan James Publishing donates one percent of all book sales for the life of each book to Habitat for Humanity. Get involved today, visit **www.HelpHabitatForHumanity.org.**

Dedication

My two sons
Hunter and Heath

These two are the real healers in my book and in my life. Even though I have spent my adult years taking care of people and have completed many years of education to be the best doctor possible, I am no match for what special healing powers my two sons possess. They are magical, and with no effort whatsoever. They have no training in healing the sick, no idea how to diagnose a condition and don't care what results blood work or x-rays show, yet their unconditional love is the best medicine in the world. I am honored to be their father and mentor as they approach the next chapter in their lives.

ACKNOWLEDGMENTS

There have been certain people in my life who have galvanized me to grow... not slowly...but with an unbridled passion and laser beam focus. These special human beings have a similar energy to mine and together, we've formed a synergy that brought about the creation of this book. I am forever grateful for their special skills, enthusiasm and love for me.

The following folks have risen far and above the level of dedication I ever expected:

Everyone needs a coach, mentor and guide to help with life's challenges. Despite how talented you may be, a good coach helps you achieve what you may never have been able to do alone. Nancy Powers has been my life coach and in my corner teaching, training, conditioning and strategizing on how to claim a victory in this boxing match of life. No one should be without a coach!

Since seventh grade, my life long friend, Carlos Castellanos has been working on projects with me. Our friendship is complete with the most memorable experiences whether it was running for high school class president or more recently striving for a global healthcare shift in consciousness with me, he is part of my family, or as he would say, "familial!"

I've been trained to believe that "there are no accidents," yet it is still quite fascinating that a complete stranger can suddenly step into your life and bridge the gap between wandering aimlessly through writing your first book and showing you the "yellow brick road." Anne Akers, the owner of MD Publish, has been my "good fairy" and every time I click my red running sneakers together, she appears with the most beautifully elegant and stately prose, that I am transported to the land of book publishing Oz.

What in the world would I have done without Paul Buckin? He started out as a patient, then a friend, then my savior during one of the toughest times of my life. Every person or animal that he meets loves him! His superior intelligence comes complete with what I refer to as "editing freakishness." He spots EVERY misspelled word, grammatical error and instances of improper syntax. He's not autistic, but he is my "Rainman" of the literary world.

How fortunate I am to have a patient and friend who is also the producer of ESPN news radio. Beth Faber is the talented person who also happens to be representative of the audience I choose to appeal to most —Moms and those that are athletically-minded. Beth has been the "fuel to my fire" as she cheered from the sidelines with comments of what makes up a superstar athlete. She has always believed that the public deserved to know the good side of professional athletes and their collective healthy habits. Despite her rigorous schedule, she still found time to assist me with interviewing tips and also which stars were most deserving and appealing.

Having appeared together on Home Shopping Network some 13 years ago, Mindy McCortney was the perfect show host. Since I also was a part of this network for awhile, she and I became friends and then ultimately book collaborators. She reviewed my first manuscript and within 24 hours, had questions and suggestions. Mindy also fits the image of my target audience as a single parent of two teenage boys. She's a voracious reader and her ideas were compelling as a "family healthcare decision maker."

Kevin O'Neill, one of the most highly respected head athletic trainers in the National Football League. After being with the Dallas Cowboys, he came to the Miami Dolphins and has been one of my favorite friends for the past 12 years. He is revered by his fellow trainers in and out of the NFL as highly intelligent, extremely conscientious, a great communicator, very diplomatic and open minded. He scoured through this book making sure there were no scathing comments, sensationalized stories or inappropriate "secrets" prepared for the "media game." His opinion and guidance has been priceless in this book and in my life – it's evidenced by his amazing children.

Every wonderful book has an amazing editor, Dr. Mara Schiff. Yet, not every wonderful book has a serendipitous story behind the discovery of its editor. Dr. Schiff, the ideal candidate, had been literally sitting in front of me for years as a patient. Not only was she a patient, but she was the creator of a book club that I was fully immersed in. One day when none of the other members showed up for our book review, we talked about our goals and I described the ideal editor and she said, "that's me!" Even though Mara had only worked on text books, she emailed a fresh sample of her writing to my book agent and it was love at first byte (megabyte).

Rene Harte had nothing to do with the writing of this book, nor the inspiration of its completion. More importantly, though, the partial owner of five comedy clubs believed in and adopted the nutritional and the physical aspects of my teachings and promptly lost 30 pounds. Her excitement began to bring this book alive and with her extreme creativity, ingenuity and passion for what we now call, "The Energy Tour," a new era has begun in my life. We've already commenced to the 50 city, education and entertainment performance platform that has enthralled and motivated all who experience it. I can't thank her enough for her faith, confidence and belief in me.

It's been 30 years since this woman was in my air space but it feels as if it was yesterday. Kathryn Lorusso is not only a highly intelligent former journalist and current high school guidance counselor, she is an extremely avid nutritional and exercise enthusiast and my best friend. She has flavored my writing with a most smooth and eloquent flow and when someone can turn my artwork into a masterpiece, they've got my attention... big time.

Joy Baron ... hmm, a little unusual for an ex-husband to express appreciation to his ex-spouse but Joy's influence on the book went a lot further than being a good mother to our children. Even though our divorce unfolded as this book was being written, she showed compassion for the process and because of that some of the most important aspects described in the book were able to develop. I am grateful for her continuing help and influence with the two little men who mean the world to me.

Lucy Unsworth is responsible for the proverbial "icing on the cake" - the cover of this book. Her skills go way beyond photography and encompass creativity, thoughtfulness, communication, and sincerity. She willingly took charge of the visual side of the book and showed the flexibility and freedom to allow anything to happen. The real beauty is what I observed behind the camera (not in front of it). Her exterior is as gorgeous as her interior is uniquely special. It takes an emotionally connected, insightful and optimistic individual to pull off a successful cover shoot.

Above all, I am happiest to know my mother is still here to read this book. Her unconditional love and commitment to her children and grandchildren are the reasons I've made it my mission to inform the public of the most powerful healing habits behind the locker room doors of America's superstar athletes.

And to all the professional athletes, doctors, athletic trainers, healthcare providers and coaches who have been mentioned in this book and have dedicated themselves to the advancement of the "new mainstream" of health awareness, I thank you with all of my heart.

Contents

Introduction

WHY ARE WE HERE?

In Other Words, Who Is Dr. Spencer Baron? And Why Should I Believe Anything He Says?

Pssst ... Hey you ... Yeah, you ... over there, come here; I want to tell you something.

It's about my secret love affair, and I want to introduce you to her.

Actually, she's not just my own. I hear similar stories from many professional athletes who have also fallen under her spell and now chase the same allure that I do.

OK, so maybe it's not so secret. Considering how much time I'm away from home satisfying my passion, you'd have to be pretty much blind to miss it. And every time I'm with her, I'm on an emotional rollercoaster; I go from joy to anger to frustration to deep love, and I've been with her over twenty years now. My former wife knows about it; my kids know; all my friends know. Now I'm about to share her with you, too.

No, she's not some hot, sexy, young blonde on whom I'm fixated. Instead, my deepest love is my fascination with health management and preventive medicine. And I'm far from alone in my fascination. Indeed, the world has also become preoccupied with this fixation on improving health through eating better, exercising more, and including nutrition and vitamins in the diet. In addition, the three thousand-year-old healing art of acupuncture and the manipulation of muscles and bones through chiropractic and massage have also become standard treatment methodologies. And then there are lasers, oxygen chambers, biomechanical evaluations under high-speed photography, specialized psychologies, sophisticated blood analysis, and even the resurrection of grandma's home remedies.

You may have dabbled with a few of these alternatives. Maybe your doctor has, too. Maybe you've never heard of any of them. Maybe your doctor hasn't, either. As the world simultaneously shrinks in size and grows in its need for a way to treat the planet's crushing health problems, some alternative treatments are becoming more mainstream, while their previously popular "traditional medicine" standbys are falling into disuse after years of inefficacy and lackluster results.

What has happened is that American healthcare is waging a battle—with itself. This "battle" is between two prevailing belief systems: traditional western medicine versus new ideas about holistic wellness. It is a battle that has been raging for decades, and it is not being fought on the battlefield by huge battalions or armored divisions, but rather in the corporate boardrooms of hospitals, pharmaceutical companies, and health insurance companies. If we are lucky—no, not lucky but *smart*—curious, health-conscious individuals like yourself, one informed consumer at a time, will ultimately win the battle.

Whether you realize it or not, you are the product of years of traditional medicine, sired on decades of sitting in your family doctor's waiting room, staring at Norman Rockwell prints of white-coated physicians bearing stethoscopes around their necks and lollipops in their pockets. Unfortunately, these doctors have also been educated, for better or worse, in a treat-the-symptoms-not-the-cause mentality that has cost you thousands of dollars in medical bills—and untold months of potential wellness. This form of medical care definitely has its place and has made enormous contributions to increasing the health and well-being of the vast majority of the population. However, traditional western healthcare may be unintentionally, and systematically, dismembering you limb by limb.

In this view of medicine, your body is seen as a system of disparate parts to be independently treated and "cured." For example, if your head hurts, you take an aspirin to dull the pain rather than seek what may be the underlying cause of that headache, such as tension from an unhealthy lifestyle, dehydration, or lack of sufficient vitamins and minerals in your diet. For examples of how prevalent this is in our current culture, consider the stream of commercials you saw when you watched television last night. You could take one medication to treat your insomnia, but it may simultaneously cause impotence, stomach upset, and dizziness. While another prescription may help your gastritis, it concurrently causes an ulcer, migraine headache, or insomnia. You can take one pill to lower your blood pressure, another to treat your elevated cholesterol, and yet another to control your psoriasis, but each of these will potentially cause some new problem requiring some additional treatment. Each new "cure" creates some other illness, requiring some other drug to treat it. Your body is cut into disconnected pieces as individual components are examined and treated. When does it end? At what point do we say, "Enough!" and start treating our bodies as the extraordinary, self-healing, and unified mechanisms they are designed to be?

DR. BARON'S SUPERSTAR HEALTH TIP:

Our current treat-the-symptoms-not-the-cause mentality has cost you thousands of dollars in medical bills—and untold months of potential wellness.

One arena that has seen amazing advances in how to respond to and treat the human body is the world of professional sports. A professional athlete's body is a finely tuned machine, required to consistently operate at peak capacity in order to command the millions of dollars the athlete receives in salary and endorsements. An athlete's body does not belong to him or her alone. It also belongs to the team that pays for and depends on it. It belongs to the companies that invest in it and will receive millions of dollars from the product sales it generates. It belongs to the public who spend thousands of dollars each year to watch it. It is a *moneymaking machine.*

Not only are millions of dollars made from this high-powered machine, but equal amounts are invested in keeping it healthy and functioning at peak performance. Coaches, athletic trainers, team doctors, yoga and meditation masters, acupuncturists, and herds of others are employed to keep professional athletes functioning at their best, all the time. No one makes a nickel if the player can't play. No one wants to watch a tired, bruised, and battered competitor dragging his way onto the field for another painful round. The world of professional sports is often on the cutting edge of new treatments and therapies designed to keep its athletes functioning at top physical, mental, and nutritional capacity.

DR. BARON'S SUPERSTAR HEALTH TIP:

The body of a professional athlete is a moneymaking machine, and millions of dollars are invested in keeping it functioning at top mental, physical, and nutritional capacity.

So, how does this relate to you?

Well, you have an important decision to make. Are you willing to open your mind to new and alternative ideas about health, medicine, and your overall well-being that come from the world of professional sports and its multimillion-dollar investment in the health and well-being of its players? Are you willing to consider how these top secret treatments, cures, and principles may be able to work for you and your health?

Your health is your most important asset. In traditional health care, you entrust your care to others who, you believe, know what is best for you and who, you believe, are operating in your best interest. Your doctor, your health insurance company, and the drug companies are all trying.

Consider for a moment that this may not be true. The information provided to you by others may be tainted with their own values, biases, and self-interests (read: *profit*) that may not be consistent with your own. In professional sports, however, everyone has the same interest—making money off the players. That can only happen when the players are in top shape and operating under the care and guidance of trained health-care professionals who, let's face it, also profit from the well-being of their athletes.

And that is where you have a decision to make.

You are your own best advocate and the best person to make decisions about your life, your body, and your health. But this is only true *if* you are well informed about your choices, your body, and the possibilities available to you for self-care and healing.

DR. BARON'S SUPERSTAR HEALTH TIP:

Your health is your most important asset. You are the best person to make decisions about your life, your body, and your health, but only *if* you are well informed about your choices, your body, and the possibilities available to you for self-care and healing.

The purpose of *Dr. Spencer Baron's Secrets of the Game* is to introduce you to a new possibility—the idea that you can have the extraordinary health and fitness of a superstar athlete without the million-dollar price tag. Health is an equal-opportunity resource; it is there for the taking, if only we will shake off the fog of traditional medicine's "treat-the-symptoms" mentality and open our eyes to the possibility of having all the *Secrets of the Game.*

Who Is Dr. Spencer Baron? And Why Should You Trust Me?

So why should you believe anything I say? Before I launch into my professional background that qualifies me to write this book and to give you advice on your own health and well-being, I want to share a story with you. This story is important because, although it happened a long time ago, it made me who I am and set me on a lifelong path dedicated to healing others.

In 1977, I was a recovering nerd wearing thick, black, plastic glasses with shockproof lenses, sporting a bushy white-boy Afro on my feeble 127-pound frame. Having spent much of my youth fighting to defend myself and most of my geeky, outcast friends, I was a remarkably good fighter, despite my unseemly appearance. When I discovered wrestling, my whole life changed.

In eleventh grade, I became a high school wrestling sensation. In October of that year, I was a sixteen-year-old, hotshot wrestler competing in a preseason qualifying tournament. My third match of the evening appeared to be another easy win with an advance to the semifinals. I was up two points and nearing the end of the second two-minute round. While my awkward opponent held me in a headlock, I felt a subtle snapping in my neck; the discomfort was dulled, however, by the adrenaline and anticipation of victory. After the match, I mentioned the mild discomfort to Coach Frayer, who suggested I forfeit the tournament rather than risk getting injured. Of course, my teenaged belief in my own invincibility sent me straight back onto the mat.

In the third and final round, I was mildly stiff but immensely determined. I was behind by one point and ready to take my opponent down. On both feet, facing my adversary and ready to lunge like a starving tiger, I went in for the takedown. Suddenly, both arms got tied up, as I tripped over my opponent's foot with nothing to brace my fall. I landed on my head and, as I went tumbling down, I heard a sickening CRACK that sounded like a dry branch snapping in a quiet forest. As I crumbled to the mat, the coach, the team, the referee, and the spectators knew something was gravely wrong.

Through the searing pain, I could hear Coach say to me, "Move your fingers ... How 'bout the toes?"

I somehow successfully passed the test and got up, despite the sensational pain that accompanied every breath. The long drive home was torturous, as my parents waited tensely by the front door.

Desperate to calm my overanxious mother, I continued to try to suppress the pain throughout that night. I was sure aspirin and an electric heating pack would do the trick but, by morning, the pain had worsened significantly, and my parents worriedly drove me to the hospital. I thought my head would explode from the pain of that drive.

After several X-rays and the medical doctor's evaluation, there were still no answers. My parents and I were terrified of what awful news the doctor might deliver as we sat, exasperated and bewildered, bracing ourselves for the worst and hoping for the best. We unquestioningly trusted the all-knowing doctor.

Finally, the doctor reappeared. "We need to check in the patient," he said. "We still don't know what's wrong, but we want to keep him in traction and under surveillance." The next thing I heard blew me away. "There is too much muscle development around his neck, and we are unable to determine if there is a fracture or not."

Wow, I thought, *that's actually kinda cool*. Too much muscle? I'd never heard *that* associated with *me* before. However, as the reality set in and I realized I was going to miss a week of school and, more importantly, wrestling practice, the glow began to dim.

The pain began to improve, although I was unsure whether that was because the medication was dulling the discomfort or actual healing was occurring. As friends visited the hospital, there was not much time alone to dwell on the problem. (I'll never forget Fran, my dream girl, sauntering through the door. She was tall, supercool, and beautiful—someone who would *never* like me. When she leaned over to kiss me goodbye, I could almost bear the searing pain that threatened to overwhelm my body. It *truly* was worth it!) I was released after a week in traction with still no answers as to what happened to me. Moreover, I would now have to spend the next three months confined to a hard, plastic neck brace—a daunting prospect for a young, active kid.

When I was allowed to walk again, I stumbled back to be part of my team. With a rigid cervical collar protecting every head movement, my participation was limited to supportive cheers from the sideline as my teammates smacked down their opponents. I sullenly watched the guy who took my place immersed in the "thrill of victory." Good sportsmanship notwithstanding, for me, it was really the "agony of defeat."

Over time, the physical pain eased, but the emotional anguish became intractable. I cried alone almost every night as I felt stripped of my most wondrous privilege—the opportunity to compete and win in a sport and to escape the miserable prospect of being a 98-pound, weakling dork forever. As a teenager, my identity and self-esteem were all wrapped up in my wrestling success, and I felt undeservedly robbed of my dreams. I have never quite lost the feeling of being that poor, despondent kid feeling destined to the life of a misfit.

When I sit across from a patient faced with a debilitating injury, I am transported to that childhood bed in the dark and my own secretly wept tears. It doesn't matter if he is a world-class athlete or she is a mom who can no longer pick up her youngest daughter because of her pain. It has become my deepest passion to heal my patients' injuries by using use all of the principles I have dedicated myself to learning since that event. I am 100 percent committed to making that person better. I *know* I can do it, and with the right health-care team, it can happen faster and more efficiently than most of the health-care professionals out there can make it happen.

In my practice, we see patients every day who are faced with similar conditions to the one I sustained as a teenager, but we can get them better in a week or two and, more importantly, give answers and a prognosis that allows them back into regular activity almost immediately. As a result of that adolescent trauma, I discovered my life's mission—to serve and empower others to heal themselves through better, more efficient, and powerful health care.

My Professional Credentials

I went on to dedicate my life to health and healing. I knew traditional medicine was not the path for me, so I enrolled in and subsequently graduated from Texas Chiropractic College in 1985. I continued my postgraduate training and became a Diplomate of the American Chiropractic Board of Sports Physicians, which has only certified 211 such doctors in the entire world.

With this specialty certification in sports injuries, I became the chiropractic consultant to the Miami Dolphins football team and the Florida Marlins baseball team, for which I both still serve. I was subsequently requested to be the chiropractor to Barry University, as well as to treat the Nebraska Cornhuskers, the New York Mets, the San Francisco Giants, and the Colorado Rockies. I am currently the president of the Professional Football Chiropractic Society, a professional organization consisting of all the chiropractors representing each of the thirty-two NFL teams. Until selling my practice in 2007, I had a thriving chiropractic office in Miami, Florida, wherein I treated hundreds of patients of all sizes, shapes, and colors, including, but not limited to, professional athletes.

I was president of the Council on Sports Injuries and Physical Fitness of the Florida Chiropractic Association from 1990 to 1992 and was Director of Sports Injuries for the Dade County Chiropractic Society for six years. In 1993, the American Chiropractic Association Sports Council chose me to serve as the delegation leader to a team of eighteen sports chiropractors in an educational exchange with the Sports Medicine Physicians of the National Chinese Olympic Training Center in Beijing, China. In 1992, I became the first on-staff chiropractic physician at Doctors Hospital of Hollywood, a position newly created for me and unparalleled in any other hospital throughout the country. In 1994, I was designated head of the department for the Chiropractic Division with Golden Glades Regional Medical Center.

Some of the most gratifying moments in my 18-year career have been spent treating the casts of *CATS*, *Crazy for You*, *Les Misérables*, The Rockettes, *Jesus Christ Superstar*, *West Side Story*, *Damn Yankees*, *Chicago*, and *Celtic Fusion*, as Broadway shows have begun seeing the extraordinary virtue of using chiropractic to treat their cast members.

Why This Book and Why Now?

So why should you believe me?

The answer is: *You shouldn't.*

There is only one way you will know if I am worth my salt. Try for yourself and see if the treatments, therapies, and lifestyle suggestions I offer in this book make a difference for you. I am absolutely certain that I can enhance your life, as I have done for countless others—athletes and nonathletes alike. The fact of the matter is that, simply by picking up this book and reading it, you are already on your way to the best health of your life. But don't just take my word for it.

DR. BARON'S SUPERSTAR HEALTH TIP:

You are already on your way to
the best health of your life!

If you are already in your best shape ever, and you believe there is nothing else for you to learn, then great. But if you are not, I invite you to consider some new possibilities that may not fit into your "box" of what you think is the best and most appropriate health care for you. Even though I have suggested that you don't trust me, I am going to ask you to trust the ideas and therapies I present in this book—not because you know me personally and can attest to my trustworthiness but because I have helped thousands of people experience their lives and their bodies in unprecedented ways.

The rest of this book is devoted to a few simple, yet effective, ideas. First, I want to share with you how our current health care went from Point A to Point B—that is, how the history of Western medical practice developed in such a way that you have been systematically trained to believe that a particular brand of care is the right, best, and only way to go. Yes, I'm sorry, but you have been a bit manipulated. Well, not a bit … a lot. Read it and weep, my friends. (By the way, if you think this historical journey might *bore* you to tears instead, you have my permission to simply trust me and jump into the "meat" of the strategies; you can skim chapters 1, 2, and 3 and jump right on into chapter 4 on "Secrets of the Mind."

Second, I want to show you some low-cost physical, mental, and nutritional approaches to getting healthy and staying healthy—strategies that America's superstars utilize behind the scenes. I want to offer you insights into how "A-list" athletes have achieved their success, how they maintain their drive and ambition, and, most importantly, how they continuously push their bodies and minds to extreme limits—quite successfully.

Finally, I want you to see for yourself what some of these amazing athletes and the teams of professionals employed to keep them in top shape say about the strategies I present to you in this book. You will read quotes from these individuals regarding how to achieve your goals, whatever your goals may be, and how to become a "superstar" in your own life. The tools are here; you decide if, when, and how you want to use them.

The idea is simple. You must be willing to let go of some of your old ideas and old ways of thinking in order to let some new information in. The results will eventually speak for themselves.

So, put on your literary running shoes and let's get moving!

DR. BARON'S SUPERSTAR HEALTH TIP:

You must be willing to let go of some of your old ideas and old ways of thinking in order to let some new information in. The results will eventually speak for themselves.

Chapter 1

THE BATTLE OF BELIEF

Athletes have gotten smarter, better with nutrition and rest, more attuned to what their bodies need. That awareness has become greater over years gone by as heightened awareness in society has facilitated this perspective. Whereas, maybe thirty years ago, a guy got injected and was told, "You're playing this week." this approach is not taken anymore, anywhere.
Kevin O'Neill, Miami Dolphins Head Athletic Trainer

Did you know that the first surgeons were actually *barbers*? Yep, that's right—the kindly old man who trims your hair and beard in a chair with a candy-striped pole out front, once was also the guy who removed your appendix, pulled your teeth, and stemmed your internal bleeding. Until the mid 1700s, it was commonly held that barbers could perform amputations; remove odd, external growths; and perform other surgical feats. The absence of anesthesia and sterilization was directly related to the amount of blood lost and trauma suffered. Here's a little-known fact: You know where that symbolic candy-striped pole came from? It is derived from the blood and bandages that would hang out to dry by the barber-surgeon's shop. Yikes! You'll never look at one of those quite the same, will you?!

This notion of the barber-surgeon was the genesis of Western medicine's outpatient care model. Did you ever stop and wonder what happened to the doctor who used to make house calls and take care of your *whole* body? Today, we call them "general practitioners," but even these guys are becoming obsolete in the world of highly specialized care. If your foot hurts, you go to a "foot doctor," known as a podiatrist; if your shoulder joint hurts, you go to an orthopedist, who takes care of bones and joints; the neurosurgeon handles your brain and spinal cord. When you have a pain in the butt, you go to your proctologist (or the corner bar!), and so on. This medical model is known as *allopathic medicine*, in which disease is identified as a set of symptoms that can be isolated from other body parts and functions and then independently treated. For example, you get treated for chronic pain in the shoulder blade (scapula) nearest to the spine, only to find out the origin of the problem is in your gallbladder, which remained untreated because it hasn't been identified as or even linked to the cause of the problem in your scapula. We call this "referred pain," and it can be a tricky symptom if not properly diagnosed.

In contrast to practitioners from the Western hemisphere, who focus on a *mechanistic body* paradigm, wherein the body operates as a slick machine composed of independent parts, practitioners from Eastern, or Oriental, traditions advocate a holistic approach to healing, in which the mind and body are mutually dependent. In this paradigm, each individual body component is essential to the body's overall capacity to function and heal from illness and injury. In our culture, practices associated with this latter paradigm are generally referred to as *alternative medicine*.

DR. BARON'S SUPERSTAR HEALTH TIP:

Western practitioners focus on a *mechanistic body* paradigm; Eastern practitioners advocate a *holistic mind-body* approach to healing.

This divergence of opinion between "traditional" medicine and "alternative" healthcare continues to clash, perhaps even more fervently than ever. But, before I get ahead of myself, let me offer you a brief course in Western versus Eastern Medical Philosophy 101 to bring you up-to-date how on we arrived at the set of beliefs that currently dominate our healthcare approach. Please bear with me; while this may seem like a tedious trip into historical trivia (though I promise to entertain along the way), for you to benefit fully from the concepts I present in this book, it is essential that you understand why you believe what you do, how you have been systematically trained to think *exactly* that way, and why you are powerless to change unless you see how you may have been manipulated.

Now pay attention because this is important: **NOTHING I SAY HERE IS "THE TRUTH."**

Everything I suggest in the following pages is simply a *possible way of understanding* how the world of health care works. I am recommending that you "try on" the perspective I am presenting—you *always* have the choice to take what works for you and leave what does not. If I communicate one simple message to you as you read this book and nothing else, it is this: YOU HAVE A CHOICE.

And don't you *ever, ever* let anyone tell you differently.

DR. BARON'S SUPERSTAR HEALTH TIP:

You *always* have a choice about your own health care.

A Brief History of Western Medicine

While the barber-surgeon may have been responsible for the original "cut-and-paste" model of healthcare, in 1616, a medical doctor in England named William Harvey further dissected the body's component parts, focusing on the role of blood in the body. Harvey first understood and popularized the concept of a central circulatory system (like a computer's primary "operating system," for all you PC and MAC users) that pumped blood into and through the heart.

His insight was the first to begin redirecting practitioners' thoughts away from the traditional practice of bloodletting as a cure for disease toward an understanding that blood flow was essential for circulation and, thus, for the body's ability to function. Bloodletting was the practice of cutting open a vein to allow blood to drain out of the body, with the expectation that eliminating the "bad" blood would eliminate the "bad" disease. Sounds preposterous, right? Well, before Harvey's groundbreaking discovery of the importance of blood and the circulatory system, bloodletting was quite standard.

While Harvey's experiments considered how body parts and organs could be isolated and treated, he was, nonetheless, at this time still practicing within an overall context of the body as an integrated and interdependent unit. Mind and body had still not been completely severed. Awarded much merit on his mechanistic approach to the body, and consistent with the "Cartesian philosophy" (after philosopher and mathematician Rene Descartes, whom we will discuss in more detail later) that informed most scientific practice, he dismantled the body like Mark Martin's pit crew during a Daytona 500 race.

In this pre-seventeenth century world, mind and body were still linked in an overall model, wherein mental, physical, social, and environmental factors were considered equally essential to overall health and well-being. Prior to the seventeenth century, medical practice was based on the philosophy that the mind and the body were fundamentally linked and, thus, mental processes influenced physical outcomes, and physical symptoms were related to mental conditions.

DR. BARON'S SUPERSTAR HEALTH TIP:

Prior to the seventeenth century, the mind and body were fundamentally linked in health-care treatment models.

<u>Pre-seventeenth Century Beliefs</u>

MIND   BODY

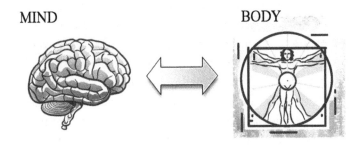

Up until about the eighteenth century, the health-care world viewed the body as a fully functioning and integrated organism. Homeopathy, a therapeutic model designed to treat the *whole* patient, was the widespread and standard treatment system of choice. This model contends that disorder and disease are expressed as a complex "collision" of events that result in physical, as well as emotional and/or mental, symptoms. Thus, body parts may not be independently isolated and *all* components need to be treated concurrently.

Louis Pasteur's "Germ Warfare"

One of the most rigorous debates in health care occurred during the nineteenth century, when Louis Pasteur, the famous microbiologist best known for establishing the relationship between germs and disease, battled it out with renowned physiologist Claude Bernard. Under Pasteur's view, disease was caused by particular microbes. From his perspective, one single and predominant factor—a germ—caused disease, rather than a constellation of physiological, emotional, and dietary factors that *simultaneously* affected the human body. The medical profession swiftly accepted this idea. You might think of it this way: if you have rats in your house, rather than cleaning up the food, throwing out the garbage, plugging up the holes, or buying a cat, you just kill the rat, and the problem disappears.

Pasteur was not only revered as an outstanding scientist, but he was also a skilled and vigorous debater with a flair for dramatic presentation.

He presented his viewpoint with such charismatic panache that it was easy to get others to accept his ideas. (He would have made a great Super Bowl commercial!) Interestingly, while Pasteur's ideas have much merit and have dominated the health-care treatment "debate" for centuries, he boldly suggested in later writings that mental states *can* affect resistance to infection. Indeed, he ultimately validated the "mind/body" connection he initially disregarded. As a result, his legacy eventually corroborated homeopathic belief.

On the other hand, Claude Bernard advocated that illness was a disruption in the fine balance between external, or environmental, factors and internal body dynamics. Specifically, Claude Bernard first described how the body possesses control systems, or *thermostats*, which will adjust to exchanges with its surrounding environment. That is, the body compensates for *signals* it receives from external conditions. To ensure that the body remains in a constant state of equilibrium, or health, this thermostat will regulate the only thing it can control: its internal physical environment.

Here is an example of how this works, though, in this case, not necessarily to your benefit. Ever heard a story of someone who went to the doctor for a routine checkup and was told he had a cancerous tumor raging in his body that would require immediate treatment—or, worse yet, that the condition was not treatable and the patient should prepare for the worst? The devastated patient then wondered, *How is this possible? I felt nothing; there was no pain at all!* This is because we can have cancer cells or other infectious diseases brewing within us at any time and never know it because our immune system, or thermostat, has been working hard to fight the intrusion and keep us healthy and strong. The patient felt a little tired, but that was all (rather like Lance Armstrong describes his experience with cancer in his bestselling memoir *It's Not about the Bike: My Journey Back to Life*).[11]. Well, the tiredness resulted because, while the body's immune system was working in overdrive to keep the body functioning and "healthy," it was actually overcompensating to fight the body's disease. While this is not the most optimistic example I can provide, it is perhaps the most dramatic and shows how amazing your body truly is.

---

1   [1] Lance Armstrong, *It's Not about the Bike: My Journey Back to Life* (USA: Penguin Group, 2001).

DR. BARON'S SUPERSTAR HEALTH TIP:

Your body has a self-regulating thermostat that will always try to maintain equilibrium.

Cartesian Philosophy and Reductionistic Theory

Enter René Descartes (1596–1650) from left field. A historic French mathematician, philosopher, and physiologist, *not* a medical doctor, Descartes first questioned the relationship between the mind, the brain, and the nervous system. While the great philosophical distinction between mind and body in Western thought can be traced to the Greeks, it was René Descartes who first suggested the mind/body relationship by identifying the pineal gland (located in the skull at the base of the brain) as the physiological location where the soul and the body intersected. His intention was not to deny the connection between the mind, body, and soul, but rather to explain and understand these in scientific terms. However, the unintended result was ultimately to disenfranchise the mind from its affiliated body.

Cartesian philosophy was the first to begin dissecting injury and illness down to its physiological cellular level. This led to use of the term "reductionistic theory" to describe the process of breaking something down further and further into its smallest component parts. As the effects of the body became increasingly separated from the mechanisms of the mind, ailments were progressively forced into being either physical or mental, but not both.

Over time, Cartesian philosophy became synonymous with reductionistic theory. While seemingly insignificant at the time, indeed this belief system permanently changed the face of modern medicine. It began the irreversible journey away from the historical mind/body connection into the now ubiquitous model where all physiological phenomena can and must be explained scientifically and where *specialized medicine* for individualized body parts dominates the health-care landscape.

Today, reductionistic thinking demands that physicians diagnose and label a disease as either physical or mental but not, heaven forbid, as both. Patients then begin to feel as though their disease must be one or the other; for chronic pain sufferers whose doctors cannot name and diagnose the source of their pain, the fallback position becomes the *other* culprit—that inexplicable, notorious, and uncontrollable mind.

DR. BARON'S SUPERSTAR HEALTH TIP:

By the seventeenth century, reductionistic theory began to separate mind and body when treating disease; this approach continues to dominate modern medicine.

Seventeenth Century: René Descartes' Cartesian Philosophy

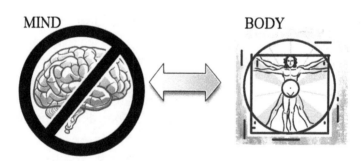

MIND   BODY

Medicine Meets Politics

In 1806, the world of health care in the United States was changed forever when a small but highly politicized group of health-care practitioners created "licensing laws." These new laws required that "medical doctors" must be licensed by the government; anyone caught practicing "medicine" without such a license could face either fine or imprisonment or both. Remember that "medicine" at this time was a vague and varying concept that included bleeding, purging, blistering, and poisoning patients with mercury—among other "scientific" treatments.

Though disguised as an effort to standardize and thus ensure the safety of medical practices, the regulation of "medicine" was *not* entirely intended to produce better, more consistent, or more reliable health care. Rather, it was expected to limit the number of practitioners able to treat patients, in a capitalistic endeavor to reduce supply, increase demand, and thus increase profit. By limiting the number and type of persons allowed to treat illness, "doctors" would become the sole source of legal treatment available to citizens who had previously been able to seek effective variety of treatment in the form of hydrotherapy, eclectics, Indian Medicine, homeopathy, herbalism, midwifery, osteopathy, chiropractic, naturopathy, a regular physician, or any combination of these. In 1847, these medical doctors united to form the American Medical Association, a powerful political lobby that would dominate, determine, and direct the face of healthcare into the twenty-first century.

This regulation became the genesis of *specialized medicine* as we now practice it. So, what becomes apparent is that this style of health-care delivery was not borne out of a desire to provide better or more efficient treatment; rather, it was a political maneuver to ensure increased profit for individual physicians with unique and specialized training.

Eighteenth and Early Nineteenth Centuries: Cartesian Philosophy and Reductionistic Theory

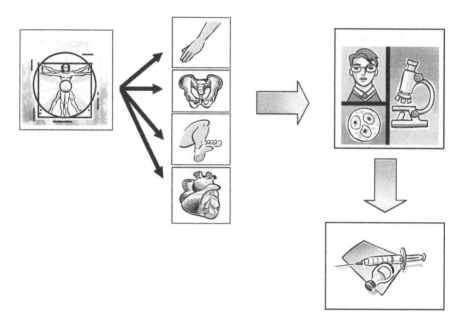

So, to summarize, what we now call "scientific medicine" has become the tendency to reduce body parts to their smallest identifiable unit to understand how each one functions individually. This has been legitimized and venerated as the highest and best practice, not because of its inherent scientific merit, but rather because a small group of smart, savvy, and politically astute observers (doctors) realized that they could profit from organizing health-care provision as a capitalistic venture.

DR. BARON'S SUPERSTAR HEALTH TIP:

The American Medical Association was originally designed as a political organization intended to restrict access to health-care practitioners.

Unfortunately, what has been lost in this journey is the critical importance of how each organ and body part relate to and depend upon the others in order for the body to function effectively and efficiently. And at the same time, the value of a variety of types and methods of therapy in an overall scheme of holistic treatment has been diminished. This process of breaking down and rendering treatment to isolated elements is the medical version of the mechanistic, assembly-line approach that has dominated Western industry since the early nineteenth century. It's like trying to review a movie by watching all the scenes separately—and maybe even out of order.

So, now here we are, deeply immersed in a medical model that treats symptoms rather than causes and reduces the body to independent, rather than *inter*dependent, components. Having been indoctrinated to believe this is the best approach, we are left with limited choices because this "way it is" is so deeply engrained in our psyches, as well as our health-care delivery systems and the finances that support this structure (in terms of insurance, specialized doctors, and governmental regulations), that it is difficult to see what may be available outside the walls of this restricted box.

DR. BARON'S SUPERSTAR HEALTH TIP:

We are now deeply immersed in a model of specialized medicine that treats symptoms rather than causes and reduces the body to independent components.

So the critical question becomes this: What's the alternative? If this is "the way it is," what choice do I really have? Well, that is what I am here to share with you, based on my own experience working with a variety of treatment modalities, superstar athletes and athletic teams, and by sharing with you what the "experts" have to say. Before we can move forward, however, I first want to offer you another perspective on health-care history that originates in the Eastern hemisphere and that suggests another way of understanding how the body works and how best to treat it. The next chapter will offer you some insights into traditional Eastern medicine, homeopathy, and how to integrate these with Western practices within an overall strategy for optimal health.

Chapter 2

A HAPPY MARRIAGE:

West Meets East

As chapter 1 explained, the history of Western medical belief through the nineteenth century was layered with extraordinary breakthrough discoveries and a corresponding movement toward diminished access to health-care services. This exclusivity was institutionalized by the emergence of the American Medical Association in midcentury, which restricted access to all health-care providers other than licensed medical doctors who would care for patients only with agreed-upon treatments. While these developments were dominating health-care trends in the West, another movement was also gaining recognition as a viable alternative and effective form of care. This type of treatment was not based on the idea of a "mechanistic body," wherein the body was regarded as an assembly line built of independent parts; this movement saw the body as intrinsically interconnected and interdependent.

Now, I'd like to share with you an alternative version of medical history. In this version, health care addresses the body holistically;

in other words, it maintains that each system functions as a direct reflection of the health and well-being of the others, that no body part operates in isolation, and that each system depends on each of the others for optimal well-being. If one body part, system, or function is ailing, so too are all the others, and *all* need to be simultaneously addressed and cared for.

Eastern Homeopathy and Western Allopathic Medicine

A German doctor named C. F. S. Hahnemann advocated a system of medicine called homeopathic medicine. This model suggested that substances could be ingested or applied to the body to mimic the symptoms of a particular disease or condition and thus build the body's tolerance to that disease or infection. The purpose was to build up and strengthen the body's *own* ability to cure itself before the illness could overtake the body, rather than relying on the introduction of some additional substance (a drug) to cure the illness. Hahnemann coined the term *allopathy* in 1842 to distinguish his homeopathy from the more traditionally accepted Western style of medicine, which he found less effective and inefficient.

Traditional Western allopathic medicine administers a dose of some drug to reproduce the symptom of health in a person's body or, put another way, to induce symptoms different from those produced by the disease. While this sounds logical, the key word here is *reproduce*. Reproducing a symptom is not the same as actually producing it. It is mimicking something but not actually causing it.

Remember that thermostat we discussed earlier? Homeopathy uses the idea that the body's own immune system can be efficiently stimulated to achieve equilibrium or health. By administering small doses of a foreign substance, the body develops immunity to the disease-causing agent and can then tolerate the symptoms of the disease. Consider the drug addict who needs more and more of a drug over time to get high because smaller doses have less effect. The body has developed a tolerance or immunity to the foreign substance—the drug. Homeopaths use this principle to the body's advantage by producing and stimulating health rather than disease.

Hahnemann originated the term *allopathy* to differentiate a rival approach that used substances that produced the opposite of a disease's symptoms to heal people. The term *allo* is Greek for "different," while *homeo* means "the same." So, in allopathy, a drug mimics health as a means of convincing the mind that the body is indeed healthy. For example, a fever reducer mimics the feeling of health but does not address the original cause of the fever. A fever is the body's way of telling you that there is an infection somewhere and it is heating the body to, in essence, isolate and "fry" the infection and thus eliminate it. Homeopaths began using the term *allopath* in the nineteenth century as a derogatory term to describe practitioners of "traditional" medicine who used what the homeopaths believed was a limited and imperfect practice of simply treating symptoms.

While homeopathy did not originate in the East, it was conceptually similar to traditions used by practitioners of Chinese medicine. By relying on natural roots and herbs and considering the genesis of disease in the body's basic immune system functions, it was more consistent with Eastern than Western medical philosophy. While homeopathy became quite popular in the United States and Europe in the 1800s, it also became the object of deep-seated animosity and vigilant opposition from the traditional medical establishment. Even though its strongest advocates included European royalty, American entrepreneurs, literary giants, and religious leaders, the conflict between homeopathy and orthodox medicine was prolonged and bitter. It's pretty obvious who won the first round (at least in the United States. In Europe and the other Americas, it's quite common to see homeopathic pharmacies as often as other drugstores). The United States is coming around, however, as more comprehensive and holistic approaches to healing are becoming popular.

DR. BARON'S SUPERSTAR HEALTH TIP:

Western allopathic medicine treats individual symptoms of disease; Eastern homeopathic medicine uses holistic approaches to treat the whole body.

Here is another way to think of it: a homeopathic response to infection would be to administer minute doses of the infectious agent to the body in order to build up the body's own resistance to that agent. Consider the child who plays in the dirt, gets covered with muck, and then goes inside to eat lunch without washing her hands. While that may seem a bit gross and the child may get an unpleasant stomachache, she also may develop a tolerance for the natural muck that exists in her environment so that it may not affect her so drastically the next time. Don't misunderstand me, I am not advocating that you don't wash your child's hands before he or she eats—quite the opposite. Washing hands regularly is essential for good health, and good old soap and water are powerful tools in fighting disease and infection. However, the antibacterial washes that are all the rage have the unintended consequence of lowering our resistance to disease by thwarting our body's own ability to deal with various natural germs and microbes in our environments. A little muck may not necessarily be such a bad thing!

A typical allopathic response to infection is to kill it with antibiotics. While this may make sense on the surface, it also ignores the simple yet obvious concurrent strategies of educating the patient on the importance of washing hands, getting rest, eating nutritious foods, eliminating emotional stresses, and exercising as a means to prevent infection in the first place. From a social perspective, allopathic medicine developed as an approach to compensate for the unhealthy lifestyles that most of us are content to live. From an economic perspective, allopathic medicine generates millions of dollars for doctors, insurance providers, pharmaceutical companies, and others who profit from this form of specialized and isolated treatment. No one profits from washing hands, eating right, and getting enough sleep!

Think of it this way: if you have a headache, you take an aspirin, and your headache is gone, right? Wrong. The aspirin is simply *reproducing* the feeling of wellness. It is not actually making you well. It is covering up the feeling of the headache by blocking your body's pain receptors. The headache is still there—you simply can't feel it. If you have arthritis, allopathy treats the pain by masking the symptoms, but the arthritis itself doesn't go away. If you have high blood pressure, drugs may lower your blood pressure, but they do not alleviate the causes for your elevated blood pressure. If you stop taking the drugs, your blood pressure shoots up again. If you don't take the painkillers, your arthritis still hurts.

The type, degree, and effect of this type of medicine exist on a continuum. Cancer-fighting drugs used in chemotherapy *are* in fact attacking the disease with the goal of eliminating it. There is absolutely nothing wrong with this. The problem is that chemotherapy also attacks other healthy organisms in the body as well and makes them sick. Hair loss, nausea, immune-system deficiencies, and decreased white blood cell counts are all examples of how the cancer-fighting drugs create additional problems in the body by attacking only one area independently and ignoring the rest. Allopathic doctors must therefore prescribe additional drugs to address symptoms that emerge in other parts of the body. As disciples of Western medical tradition, we have come to accept this process as a "normal" and routine part of the cancer-fighting process.

Eastern Homeopathic and Holistic Methods

While modern allopathy treats cancer as a disease itself, homeopathic philosophy holds that cancer is, in fact, indicative of some broader systemic disorder (or dis-ease) within the body that needs to be treated. The actual *cause* of the disease is a toxic, acidic terrain in which the body's overall immune system has been congested and has allowed "bad" cells to replicate. Allopathy treats this systemic problem by chemically attacking the individual cells associated with the cancer or, sometimes, by simply cutting them out, as in recommending double mastectomies for women with breast cancer, so as to eliminate the body part in which the cancer cells manifested. Please understand, I mean no offense here to women who have chosen this course of treatment as the right one for them; I am simply using this graphic example to make my point that surgical solutions are a standard and acceptable form of treatment in allopathic care.

Homeopathy also treats "according to the symptoms" (cancer, in this case) but not by attacking. The homeopath gives the body a minute quantity of substance that provokes the body to develop its own infection-fighting capabilities. In cancer treatment, for example, a homeopath might select a remedy that matches the symptoms of the tumor itself and focus on targeting the tumor to reverse its growth. Some homeopaths might also give remedies at the tumor site itself (in the form of an injection) to more aggressively stimulate a response. A homeopath might use remedies that assist in healing the patient's eliminative channels (kidneys, urinary tract, lymphatic system, liver, and other cleansing organs) to strengthen cell detoxification. Finally, another homeopathic approach might be to address the overall constitution of the patient by doing a complete assessment of the patient's mental, emotional, and physical symptoms and then selecting the best match accordingly that will, in turn, directly affect the tumor. These may sound ludicrous to a Western-trained mind, but the key in homeopathy is to manage *all* the body's parts and thus eliminate symptoms *before* the body is overwhelmed by the problem.

In Eastern medical philosophy, health is more than just the absence of disease and injury; rather, it refers to the optimal balance of health. When applied to health, there are three components that, together, result in *homeostasis*, or equilibrium:

1. Mental health
2. Physical health
3. Nutritional health

DR. BARON'S SUPERSTAR HEALTH TIP:

The three essential components to optimal health are mental health, physical health, and nutritional health.

Organisms and cells have the ability to maintain internal equilibrium by adjusting any one or all of these processes to adapt for dysfunctions in the others. For example, when the body ingests too much caffeine (a nutritional substance), it reacts by causing the nerves to become hyperexcitable (a physical process), which causes overstimulation and muscle spasm resulting in what you may experience as anxiety or stress (a mental state). Or, let's say you lift heavy items at work and you injure your back (a physical symptom). The injury causes some anxiety (a mental process) as you cannot carry out tasks, have sex, sit on the toilet, or pick up dropped items. This, in turn causes poor eating habits (a nutritional effect) as you eat to compensate for your feeling of incompetence or deprivation (a mental process).

Not clear yet? Try this one: That hottie you've been dating breaks up with you, and you are devastated (a mental condition), so you lose your appetite (a nutritional symptom), which leaves you weak and tired with decreased muscle density, which results in less energy and stressed joints that cannot manage regular exercise. So, you are getting fatter and experiencing a series of strains and sprains (a series of physical symptoms). Make sense now? I would bet money you've seen something like this happen to someone you know!

Chinese (Eastern) and "alternative" health-care philosophies operate on a triangulated system that equally considers the three essential components—mental, physical, and nutritional—in understanding total health:

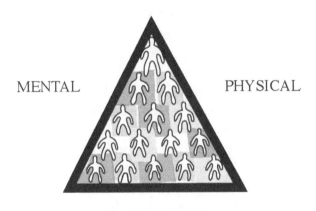

MENTAL   PHYSICAL

NUTRITIONAL

This is the foundation of traditional Chinese (Eastern) health care and what has become known in the West as "alternative" treatment philosophies. According to Eastern tradition, when effectively balanced with one another, these three elements are the fundamental keys to optimal well-being.

Reconciling the Two Perspectives

Let me share a personal story. In 1991, I was sent to the National Olympic Training Center in Beijing, China, for an educational exchange with their Asian medical doctors. While walking through the compound, I waved to a man as he rode his bicycle with one hand and held an acupuncture mannequin with the other. It was one of the Olympic team's physicians. What I saw over the next two weeks astounded me.

The primary health-care system in this impoverished country (which, by the way, placed *fourth* out of 52 countries in the 1992 Summer Olympic Games) consisted of manual therapy (spinal and joint manipulation), herbs, Tai Chi, Qui Gong (therapeutic exercises developed for health and well-being), and acupuncture. During tours of traditional Chinese hospitals, I saw acupuncture in the emergency rooms, enormous herb pharmacies, and Qui Gong. Ironically, a lowly little "American pharmacy" went pretty much unnoticed by passersby.

I was rendered speechless (and for those who know me, this is pretty remarkable!) by the practices I witnessed and by the entire health-care delivery system as I saw it practiced in China. I was so moved by this experience that I reoriented my own practice to include and reflect what I learned. Moreover, I have continued to learn and expand upon teachings I first witnessed on that trip. My personal approach has consistently been oriented around utilizing the best of both worlds (Eastern and Western) by encouraging health-care providers to work together so that they may identify the most appropriate level and type of treatment that best serves the patient—the ultimate triage. I have found that integrating these three essential components works extremely well for professional athletes, whose bodies are "hot commodities" worth hundreds of thousands or millions of dollars. Their expeditious recovery is critical, as I have witnessed extraordinary healing as a result of consistently integrating mental, nutritional, and physical modalities.

Interestingly, a recent study empirically validates my own experience and demonstrates the effectiveness of this form of health care for athletes. In 2005, a Taiwanese study examined injury management models of elite athletes. The study included 393 study subjects, who averaged around 21 years old and whose average athletic experience was just under 10 years. Interestingly, 14.5 percent chose Western treatment alone, 8.1 percent chose Chinese medicine alone, and *75.4 percent received combined treatment.* The study concluded that elite athletes preferred a combination of Eastern and Western treatments for sports injuries and suggested that, "Doctors trained in Western medicine should learn these alternative treatment methods and apply them effectively in athletes, so that a better medical network can be established."[2]

---

2   SK Chen, YM Cheng, YC Lin, YJ Hong, PJ Huang, and PH Chou PH, "Investigation of Management Models in Elite Athlete Injuries," *Kaohsiung Journal of Medical Sciences* 21(5) (2005): 220-7. Department of Orthopedics, Kaohsiung

America has come a long way, yet we still manage to miss some critical components of effective health-care delivery. Despite the fact that, according to World Health Organization statistics, the United States ranks *number one* in health-care spending, it ranks number twenty-four in health life expectancy. In comparison, Japan is number one in health life expectancy, yet the country uses less than half the amount of money spent by the United States. Something is wrong with this picture. The striking disproportion of cost versus effectiveness in the United States is startling.

Some suggest that all nonmechanistic health-care modalities are "quackery" or too "New Agey." Despite having a more than 5000-year history, much in Eastern philosophical thought is now considered "new" as it reaches Western minds in a variety of forums and formats. And, as often occurs with most "new" philosophies, there is a lack of clear definition about what *it* is; this lack results in a variety of practices and processes that fall under the umbrella of "care" and "healing," which may in fact be less than reliable. However, what is important is not whether one or the other philosophical approach is "right" or "best," but rather whether a variety of modalities can coexist under a continuum of care model and be used together to most effectively treat illness and injury. A popular fable offers a useful allegory for this perspective:

> Six blind men were asked to determine what an elephant looked like by feeling different parts of the elephant's body.
>
> The blind man who feels a leg says the elephant is like a pillar; the one who feels the tail says the elephant is like a rope; the one who feels the trunk says the elephant is like a tree branch; the one who feels the ear says the elephant is like a hand fan; the one who feels the belly says the elephant is like a wall; and the one who feels the tusk says the elephant is like a solid pipe.
>
> A wise man explains to them: All of you are right. The reason every one of you is telling it differently is because each

---

Medical University Chung-Ho Memorial Hospital, Kaohsiung Medical University, Kaohsiung, Taiwan.

> one of you touched a different part of the elephant. So, actually the elephant has all the features you mentioned.3

Thus, one animal may look different to each observer. Likewise, health care suffers from the same limitation; each perspective results in a different analysis of what *it* (disease or injury) is and, thus, limits how to treat it.

As I have suggested before, there is no such thing as *The Truth*; "truth" appropriately resides in the mind (and body) of the beholder. I hope to offer you the tools to identify what *it* is yourself and then seek the best treatment to resolve your problem. For some of you, the benefits of homeopathy will seem logical and intuitive. For others, its attributes may seem less apparent. That's fine. My job is not to convince you that one system is better than another; rather, it is to provide you with sufficient information so that you are able to make an *informed choice* about your own health-care options.

DR. BARON'S SUPERSTAR HEALTH TIP:

My goal in this book is to provide you with information to make an informed choice about your own health care.

So, now you are faced with a critical question.

How do you, as the ultimate health-care spectator, get more than just a ringside seat? In other words, how do you start actively playing *on the court* of your own health and well-being, rather than simply observing from the sidelines while others make game winning, or losing, choices and decisions for you? The fact of the matter is that the less informed you are, the more dearly you continue to pay—with substandard treatment, less medical coverage, and greater apathy from your healthcare provider.

---

3   *Wikipedia: The Free Encyclopedia*, s.v. "Blind Men and an Elephant," http://en.wikipedia.org/wiki/Blind_Men_and_an_Elephant#_note-JainWorld (accessed December 9, 2008).

Dr. Baron's Superstar Health Tip:

The less informed you are, the more dearly you pay— with substandard treatment, less medical coverage, and greater apathy from your health-care provider.

That is, until you ask yourself, "What else can I do?"

CHOICE: *The Undisputed Champion*

Often in my 21 years in practice, I have heard the same things from patients: "I don't want surgery." "I don't want medication." "I don't want to continue being injured or sick." "I've tried everything; isn't there another way?"

So many of the "specialists" my patients had seen before coming to me were, indeed, limited by their own brilliance.

Huh?

Yes, these "brilliant" doctors and other health-care professionals were limited because, while exceptionally talented, competent, and accomplished, their expertise was limited to only one area. Their very narrow views were often presented, and thus interpreted, as the "only option." Moreover, often that "only option" would offer only a short-term solution alongside what, in fact, was a long-term failure. In other words, "Give a man a hammer, and everything is a nail," wrote Mark Twain. To a surgeon, most everything is operable; to an orthopedist, most everything requires an orthopedic solution. My chiropractic colleagues and I would often marvel at the untapped array of treatments that could have safely and expeditiously restored a patient's well-being when a "traditional doctor" assured him or her that surgery was the only option.

While no one treatment is the panacea or the end-all miracle cure, typically there were multiple treatment options available that most of my patients had never even heard of, let alone considered relevant to their unique problems. Some approaches seem inaccessible because they remain very expensive. Others seem unavailable because "big business" has not done a commercial for them and thus you do not know they exist. You may have missed a treatment option due to its margin of profit, which is too low to make it widely available; or perhaps it derives from a natural resource that hasn't been bottled or packaged. Sometimes these treatments are so cutting edge that they have not hit the mainstream market yet.

The point is this: the persistent and undeniable truth in health care is that you *always, always* have a choice. To that end, I have two goals in writing this book. First, I want to broaden your knowledge and understanding of the health-care options available to you and offer you a concise and readable reference guide about those options. Second, I believe that the most impressive array of multiple strategies and methods of using them effectively are employed in treating professional athletes, for the purpose of optimizing their performance and well-being. That is, due to professional sports' underlying profit motive, the most amazing variety of health-care providers unite for the benefit of the athlete and his or her ongoing performance. I want to share those strategies.

What Does All This Mean To You?

In general, most of us tend to think of doctors, hospitals, and medicine as above repudiation and beyond reproach. And while health-care professionals, like those in law enforcement, education, and a variety of other fields, may ultimately be committed to a higher calling of service to others, medicine does not exist in a vacuum. Good health care takes money, and lots of it, just like everything else. Indeed, health care has been, and always will be, one big sales pitch. (In case you are not quite convinced, just for fun, the next time you sit down to watch television, count how many of the commercials in your favorite nighttime one-hour drama are about drugs or some other health-related topic; next time you read your favorite magazine, note how many full-page, glossy ads are devoted to drugs.) Often presented as science, a really emotional commercial, sex, or just something your "trusted" doctor tells you, what you hear, see, and feel (and sometimes smell and taste) convinces you to try the latest drug or treatment option.

DR. BARON'S SUPERSTAR HEALTH TIP:

Exploiting the best of Eastern and Western health care is, unquestionably, the best approach.

My experience and training over the years has firmly convinced me that exploiting the best of both Eastern and Western health-care worlds is unquestionably the best approach. Fortunately, and consistent with my own intuition and education, this perspective is now shared at the level of professional athletics. And the bottom line is that professional sports are all about pleasing you, the consumer, without whom there *are no* multimillion-dollar contracts and corporate support. Because of you, superstar athletes are worth millions of dollars in revenues, endorsements, and corporate sponsorship, and nobody wants to lose a dime of those profits. Therefore, expeditious recovery for athletes is critical, and preventing injury and illness in the first place is an even higher priority. What I have seen is that the constant integration of mental, nutritional, and physical modalities offers the best and most consistent road to recovery and ultimate health.

The bottom line is that if you understand this simple idea, *YOU WILL WIN.*

DR. BARON'S SUPERSTAR HEALTH TIP:

Superstar athletes get the best care because the world of professional sports spends millions of dollars are spent to keep them in peak performance shape. You, too, can have this level of care!

Chapter 3

THE "NEW MAINSTREAM" HEALTH-CARE ENVIRONMENT:

No Pain, No Gain? That's Insane!

A Health-Care Miracle?

As mild-mannered Matt Clement (currently a pitcher for the Saint Louis Cardinals) ambled into the training room, he asked if I could treat him. He had never received chiropractic treatment and said his mother used to get them all the time and she told him, if given the opportunity, he should get one, too. After a cursory evaluation, I went to work adjusting him.

"Good to go," I said to Matt, as he went to warm up his pitching arm. He was the starting pitcher that night. A couple of days later, the quiet 27-year-old asked for another treatment and, incidentally, mentioned that he'd felt pretty good after the last one.

Matt started coming into the training room and into my office for a couple of treatments per week, always humble and reserved. Each time, I would ask Matt if he was injured. He would say, "No, just a tune-up."

After several weeks of "tune-ups," I grew concerned and asked Matt if he was *sure* there was nothing wrong. (Many professional athletes often want to keep their injuries concealed for fear that it might affect their play time or future contract negotiations.)

Matt assured me that he was fine. This time, though, he sat up, looked me in the eyes, and said, "But, Doc, is it possible that, ever since you've been taking care of me, that I've been throwing smoke?"

"What do you mean?" I questioned.

"Well, ever since college, the fastest I ever threw a baseball was 84 miles per hour; and that was just one time, and I was fatigued for the whole rest of the week." I leaned forward, listening attentively. He went on, "I have not been able to throw that fast since, and if I come close, I'm spent for several days after. The first day you treated me, my fastest ball was clocked at 92 miles per hour."

Matt was impressed. And I was fascinated. This was the first time I'd heard a pitcher describe specific and measurable results of an adjustment with such accuracy. He went on and said, "I then pitched twelve balls at 82 miles per hour, ten balls at 84 miles per hour, eight balls at 86 miles per hour, and four balls at 88 miles per hour. That's why I keep coming back to get adjusted."

When a phenomenon occurs that seems scientifically inexplicable, it gets labeled "a miracle." While, to me, this event had a fairly simple and logical explanation, to Matt, it seemed miraculous. After all, he wondered, how could popping a couple of bones make a better pitcher?

The simple explanation was that I restored the normal motion of his spine, which allowed his nervous system to better communicate with his muscles and joints. This new "communication" enabled him to throw more consistent fastballs.

The "scientific" explanation is as follows:
Chiropractic Manual Manipulation within the vertebral column, known as the adjustment, serves to improve

biomechanical and neurological function. Mechanical nerves become stimulated, which serve to:

1)   Inhibit pain;
2)   Relax tight muscles;
3)   Improve coordination.

This occurs only when the vertebral joints allow proper movement of the whole spinal column. Relaxation of tight muscles occurs by influencing inhibitory internuerons in the anterior horn, which are alpha and gamma motor neurons.

Improved coordination from mechanical nerve stimulation helps the brain to control and coordinate movement, maintain proper balance, and control muscle tone. This occurs via the dorsal/posterior columns and the dorsal and ventral spinocerebellar tracts.

Quantifiable changes during pre and post-manipulation were documented in a recent, February 2007 study published in the Clinical Journal of Neurophysiology.

Professional Athletes as Pioneers

In many ways, professional athletes have been real pioneers when it comes to pain, injury relief, and overall physical maintenance. Pro athletes endure more pain and physical deterioration in an average week than most "mere humans" do in a year—or even a lifetime. And it's not just the pounding and pummeling taken by my NFL quarterback patients or my eight-second bull-riding professional rodeo patients. Basketball players burn more calories and stress more joints in a practice, let alone a game, than many of us do in a month of casual exercise. Baseball players—particularly pitchers or heavy power hitters—can damage or otherwise strain multiple joints every inning, not to mention a whole game. Tennis players continually harm multiple pressure points, particularly in their knees and ankles every time they get on the court. (Imagine doing the same thing on only one side of your body for most of your life as tennis or golf players do—talk about growing lopsided; that is a sure recipe for injury). Each sport comes with its share of related injuries and the potential for extreme physical deterioration and debilitation. The muscle, mental, and joint fatigue endured by professional athletes is intense.

The job description of a professional athlete includes extreme physical duress as a standard, daily practice. This ages, stresses, and strains them. Professional athletes are living laboratories for studying the effects of accelerated pain and muscle deterioration under rigorous conditions for weeks, months, and years at a time. Imagine feeling like you have aged six months in a single day. This is what such athletes experience day after day after day. It's exhausting just to think about it!

Millions and millions, even billions, of dollars in profit depend on these superstar athletes' health and well-being. A sick or injured athlete is not a profitable athlete; thus, he or she must be made well in hours, days, or perhaps weeks; healing certainly won't take months or years, like you and I may be told it will take.

Millions are spent to keep these athletes in prime working order. Attention to their treatment and care is no different than how a prize-winning racehorse would be cared for—a lot is riding (pun intended) on their success, and funding for their care is almost unlimited. Priorities go to what works; *mainstream* and *alternative* become meaningless distinctions in the world of professional athletic health care. If acupuncture can get a million-dollar pitcher back on the mound, bring on those needles! If chiropractic can return a pro running back to the field in 20 minutes instead of 20 days, crack those joints, baby—*RIGHT NOW*!

DR. BARON'S SUPERSTAR HEALTH TIP:

Millions and millions, even billions, of dollars in profit depend on superstar athletes' health and well-being. Priorities go to what works.

Discoveries in medicine or any other field are always initially considered breakthroughs—that is, however, until their use becomes so widespread that the general population comes to simply expect such benefits. Consider recent innovations in electronics, computers, the automotive industry, and many other fields in which remarkable advances are now considered "normal"—cell phones, laptop computers, and hybrid cars, for example, along with so many more. In health care as well, the distinctions between what's considered "normal" or "revolutionary" becomes increasingly vague as the demand for a given treatment becomes louder and louder.

DR. BARON'S SUPERSTAR HEALTH TIP:

Many of these "alternative" treatments cost no more than a bottle of aspirin and are as available to you as the corner drugstore.

How long will it be before the word *alternative* loses its meaning in the context of health care? That depends on a number of things, including but not limited to governmental policy, public and private health-care spending patterns and policies, insurance company decision-making, public demand, fiscal stability, and a variety of other conditions in what I call the "the health-care environment." I'll not bore you with any of these here; I don't want to digress into areas about which I am not fully informed or committed to sharing in this book. There are, however, many other resources for information on health-care policy.

However, a central factor in shifting the health-care environment is the degree to which health-care providers like myself—and professional athletes like those I treat—*demand* new and powerful health-care modalities and advocate for their use. Much of that impetus will come from how well we can translate and promote our passion for the best care from promises to real possibilities for you and your family; we'll then need to motivate you to join us and take action on your own behalf. And you should know, many of these "alternative" treatments may cost no more than a bottle of aspirin and are as available to you as the corner drugstore; rather, it is our lack of awareness that has become so expensive.

Game, Set, Match!

So, now that we have examined how and why our current health-care system is the way it is (in chapter 1) and considered the role of professional athletics in driving health-care treatment modalities, let's take out our magnifying glass and look *even closer*. Here are some front-row seats at the court on which this dramatic game is being played. This court is the health-care environment I referred to earlier, and it affects everything that happens to, for, or by you with respect to your own health care. This environment consists of the social, physical, and financial arenas in which health-care decision making occurs, and each decision has some impact, for better or worse, on *your* life. The drama being played out is all about you, your body, and how to keep optimally healthy and fit.

Sidelined by Sports, Rescued by Science

It's 1978. "The player" painfully hobbles over to the sideline, grimaces, and points to his leg. He indicates that the exquisite pain is located on the inside of his knee and that it occurred after a minor collision with another player. As his opponent fell, the player felt his opponent's shoulder ram into the outside area of his leg as something popped and burned. The player is brought back to the locker room, examined, injected with a heavy pain killer and anti-inflammatory agent, given a manly pat on the butt, and sent back to the field. WHATEVER IT TAKES!

That was the message delivered in the 1979 movie *North Dallas Forty*, one of the first Hollywood sports films to open the locker room doors to diehard sports fans and marginally interested spectators alike. The movie followed *Brian's Song* in 1971, an inspirational tearjerker about the life of Brian Piccolo, who died of embryonic cell carcinoma in 1970, and the smash blockbuster hit *Rocky* in 1976. For those of you who spent that year asleep or under a rock, *Rocky* told the story of underdog boxer, Rocky Balboa, as he rose from local club boxer to major professional superstar; it was the first sports film to win an Academy Award for best picture. *North Dallas Forty* gave new meaning to the phrase *no pain, no gain.* In those days, pain was a nuisance, and treatment a cost; players were expendable, and few realized this sad, sordid fact until it was too late.

In the *North Dallas Forty* era, athletic medical care was comparable to a M.A.S.H. (Mobile Army Surgical Hospital) unit in a locker room; many players only sought treatment when there was no alternative. In other words, only when, "Help! I've fallen and I can't get up," became a mantra did athletes receive any treatment at all in the training room. Injections, bandages, and pills—or what I call "symptomatic treatments"—were the traditional athletic remedies.

Today, however, elite athletes have become as astute as corporate CEOs in managing their most marketable commodity—their bodies—and they increasingly recognize the ultimate importance of long-term, strategic asset management. Rather than being considered "sissies," those players who take good and consistent care of their bodies are considered smart managers and shrewd operators. Today's players have learned from the legacies of their elders who have been left partially crippled or worse (consider Muhammad Ali); thus, they seek treatment proactively, not just reactively. However, the era of symptomatic or no treatment has left a long and depressing legacy in the form of former players who can barely stand, let alone walk, in their golden years.

Dr. Baron's Superstar Health Tip:

Elite athletes have become corporate CEOs in managing their most marketable commodity—their bodies—and they increasingly recognize the ultimate importance of long-term, strategic asset management.

What this means in the world of health care is that I, as a health-care provider, no longer see a player once or twice and never again.

Today, I see players regularly, regardless of what team they play for or where that team is located. Even when spring training in Florida is over and a northern team returns home, I know many players are following their proactive regimens in and out of the locker room by being proactive about their health in clinics all over the country.

Dismantling the Fire Alarm

Imagine this: You're just about to doze off to sleep; you think you smell a little smoke ... maybe you're dreaming. *Not to worry*, you think, *if there's anything really wrong, the smoke alarm will go off.* You hear no sound as you drift off into dreamland. Then the alarm goes shrieking off, blaring through the house, and you think, "I'm too tired to deal with this," as you sleepily shuffle over and shut off the system. Maybe the system even went back on again. This time, you decide to cut the wires to the main control panel. The system is set up to call the fire department, and when department calls to verify that there was indeed a fire blazing, you respond with a yawn, "Oh, don't worry; it'll be all right. I'll take care of it in the morning."

Absurd, right? Of course, you would never do something as dangerous as that.

But you know what? You do it *all the time* with your body. If pain was the alarm, and the fire was the problem causing the pain, would you simply eliminate the pain and ignore the fire so you could continue on about your day, week, *life?* This is what most of us do every day, and we are well trained by health-care companies, doctors, and insurance companies to do so. Every time you take an aspirin to eliminate a headache or an antacid to control your heartburn or a Lipitor to reduce your cholesterol, this is exactly what you are doing; you are dismantling the fire alarm that's telling you there's a fire raging within your body. You are handling a symptom without being responsible for considering what the cause may be.

The antacid works, but the heartburn and stomachache keep coming back. You don't change your diet much, your activities (or lack thereof) stay the same, and your stress level continues to escalate. Whenever you feel the pain, you grab another pill, especially now that the suggestion is escalating and the heartburn is worsening. Grab some more antacids; if TUMS don't work, get some Prilosec. If that doesn't do the trick, get a prescription for Zantac. I know people who take these pills before every meal to ward off the pain they have learned to anticipate will occur every time they eat.

THIS IS INSANE!

These drugs do work, and there is nothing wrong with taking them, but you should also understand that, in effect, all you are doing is shutting off the fire alarm. Maybe that's enough for you, but it's not a very effective long-term strategy to ensure long life and good health.

As the pain worsens, you finally go to the doctor. He or she refers you to a "good" internist who recommends an upper gastrointestinal (GI) tract diagnostic procedure. And guess what he finds? A brand new, fully loaded ulcer, complete with pus, scar, and dead tissue. And you know what the worst part of this is? You had the personal power and resources to have prevented the course your body followed.

Instead, you dismantled the fire alarm!

This analogy is not as far off as you might think.

DR. BARON'S SUPERSTAR HEALTH TIP:

Pain is our body's fire alarm; unfortunately, we have learned to disregard it unless the noise is deafening—and sometimes even then.

Pain is our body's fire alarm; unfortunately, we have learned to disregard it unless the noise is deafening—and sometimes even then. Mostly, we ignore the subtle aches and pains that wear us down and tire us out. We are too busy, have too much else to do, or have no time to stop; we keep on going and don't slow down. The cramping at our knee after a short run or the aching in our back after spring cleaning; the ringing in our ears or the blurriness in our vision; the rumbling in our stomachs; the stinging when we relieve ourselves—these are all fire alarms designed to warn us that there may be a fire raging inside. The "smoke" is an early detection system before the fire gets out of control.

Sometimes the most difficult part is simply knowing which aches and pains require care and which can be left to heal on their own.

Sometimes you simply don't know where to go or who to see to get effective relief. That's what this book is all about—empowering you to make informed choices about your health that are easily manageable and well within your grasp.

DR. BARON'S SUPERSTAR HEALTH TIP:

This book is all about empowering you to make informed choices about your health that are easily manageable and well within your grasp.

One of the problems with traditional (or mainstream) medicine is that it has built-in, self-serving principles. For example, when your family doctor offers you "free samples" of some drug he has been given by a pharmaceutical company representative, he is both giving his "seal of approval" to the drug, as well as setting you up to purchase more of it in the future. Lots of profits all around, no?

I am not suggesting your family doctor is intentionally in cahoots with the makers of all those antibiotics, inhalers, antidepressants, and histamine-blockers he or she hands you. What I *am* suggesting is that the interdependent structure of traditional medicine and pharmaceuticals has enhanced the latter's power and made it harder to swim against that tide; seeking other types of proactive care seems unnatural for most of us who are well-trained to accept western, allopathic approaches.

The point is this: we are used to taking "a pill for every ill" and have been systematically trained to believe that denying ourselves the comfort such medication offers is reckless and potentially destructive to our health. Rather, I am suggesting that consistently dismantling the fire alarm by covering up your body's most effective communication mechanisms (symptoms) with painkillers and antibiotics is considerably more reckless than paying close attention to your body and the messages it sends you. While there are certainly times when painkillers and antibiotics are necessary, in the long run, you are far better off seeking a remedy that can both prevent pain and discomfort *and* offer a long-term cure for the underlying problem.

<u>DR. BARON'S SUPERSTAR HEALTH TIP:</u>

While there are certainly times when painkillers and antibiotics are necessary, in the long run, you are far better off seeking a remedy that can both prevent pain and discomfort *and* offer a long-term cure for the underlying problem.

Pain Is Good!

When I was growing up, one of my athletic coaches had a saying: "No pain, no gain." For years, I believed that it was not a *real* sport unless it hurt and that I was not a *real* man unless I "played" until I felt something rip, tear, or pop!

Sound familiar? That's because a generation of coaches, athletes, and even parents were trained into thinking that pain was good—it meant "success." In those days, the result of pain was a touchdown or the celebratory rumble of your teammates jumping all over you with excitement; it didn't mean treatment, and it certainly didn't mean prevention. *That* was for wimps.

Since then, "no pain, no gain" has pretty much lost its meaning and its appeal. Modern coaches—most of them at least—know that pain is *not* gain; it is merely a physical symptom of something wrong in the body. It saps life and energy that you could better spent—say perfecting your fastball, clearing your hook shot, Or picking up your running speed by three-tenths of a minute. Whatever your athletic goals are, pain simply depletes your energy and undermines your strength.

I have a new saying: *"Pain is a drain!"*

DR. BARON'S SUPERSTAR HEALTH TIP:

Modern coaches know that pain is *not* gain; it is merely a physical symptom of something wrong in the body. I have a new saying: "*Pain is a drain!*"

This straightforward concept is the foundational support to the early and responsible management of injury and illness. Think of it this way: what if pain were a sound, and the sooner you heard that sound, the faster you could isolate the problem then solve it? Leaving it around simply drains and distracts you from what you are really committed to accomplishing—having your body work for and with you, not against you. Who wants that? Certainly not me, and I'm pretty sure not you either.

Well, pain does have a sound, and to ignore its message is to court disaster (yes, corny pun intended again). We often think that living pain free is the ultimate goal of our existence, but think rationally for a moment: no life is pain free; nor should it be. That's because "pain free" does not equal health, just as being "in pain" does not equate to sickness. And, what's more, the intensity of your pain may not directly correlate to the magnitude of the problem.

DR. BARON'S SUPERSTAR HEALTH TIP:

No life is pain free; nor should it be. "Pain free" does not equal health, just as being "in pain" does not equate to sickness.

These little aches and pains are not simply nuisances; they are alarms. Pain is an indicator—nothing more, nothing less; consider it the whiff of smoke that sets off your fire alarm. What I am suggesting is that we need to listen to our bodies more and our doctors less.

Please understand, I am *not* saying that your doctor is bad or wrong or negligent in any way. I *am* saying that we—you, me, and everyone we both know—need to take greater personal responsibility *both* for our symptoms (such as, pain) *and* for our subsequent actions (perhaps by not always simply trusting that your doctor always has all, or even the best, knowledge and information available for what ails you).

Listen to your pain; take advantage of it not by denying it but, instead, analyzing it, locating it, describing it, and then seeking treatment. One thing I've noticed about professional athletes is that they are almost obsessive about identifying and locating their pain. They won't come to me with "leg pain." Instead, they tell me exactly where that pain is, locating it by eye and hand and making me do the same. I have even had players go so far as to use a Sharpie marker to circle the exact point of their pain, like an *X* marking the treasure on an old pirate map.

DR. BARON'S SUPERSTAR HEALTH TIP:

Listen to your pain: analyze it, locate it, describe it, and *then* seek medical treatment.

Athletes are so specific about isolating the location of and accurately describing their pains because, to them, pain is a costly and debilitating obstacle. Perhaps more than most of us, athletes recognize that pain is a predictor of future performance. They recognize that a sore tendon this week could represent a sprain or tear next week; calculating the costs of losing field (or court or whatever) time makes seeking treatment an attractive and necessary option.

I always find it encouraging that these strong, powerful, physically impressive men and women never find pain a weakness, as so many of the rest of us have been trained to do. Rather, they consider it a reliable and accurate physical indicator of some underlying problem. They do not dismantle their fire alarms; they magnify the alarms by listening for the faintest sounds—day and night.

TAKE A HINT, FOLKS!

DR. BARON'S SUPERSTAR HEALTH TIP:

Pain is a reliable and accurate indicator of some underlying problem.

Readers, please take note. There is a difference between "good" pain and "bad" pain, which I will help you distinguish as we journey together through these pages. I have found that what separates the great, the good, and the merely average athletes is their ability to work through their pain—mentally and physically. A great athlete can differentiate between when the pain indicates that continuing one more step would be a career-wrecking mistake and when it is a brilliant opportunity to conquer impossible odds. What makes an athlete a superstar is that she can determine which pain may harken "the end" and which is simply an incentive to persevere toward a tantalizing and achievable victory.

Money Makes the World Go Around, the World Go Around

Why have many of the largest pharmaceutical companies started manufacturing vitamin, mineral, and herbal products? Is it their steadfast belief in this new "holistic" alternative treatment system?

Hardly. Pharmaceutical companies manufacture these products because five billion dollars per year in consumer out-of-pocket spending on herbal products alone was severely cutting into their profits. Sales of herbal products at the retail level increased from an estimate of 500 million dollars to approximately 5 billion dollars in 1999, more than double the amount compared to sales just two years before (Foster and Tyler 2000; Karch 1999).

There are three primary reasons why a pharmaceutical company would launch a subsidiary company to sell nutritional products:

1. The pharmaceutical industry is facing end-of-patent deadlines on many blockbuster drugs; when drug patents expire, manufacturers lose their monopolies and, thus, their market shares to competitors who can make and sell the same product at less cost.

2. There are no real blockbuster drugs currently heading down the research and development pipeline.

3. There has been a surge in the number of drugs withdrawn from the market for safety reasons. A side effect has been the financial bonanza for law firms initiating class action suits and a lot of unhappy pharmaceutical company stockholders.

I am not entirely sure why this is happening; maybe it's part of the "changing tides" of health care and people are finally realizing that what we have simply is not working, or at least that it's not operating entirely in their best interests. Perhaps this is the opening for a bold new era of what I call the *new mainstream*, which I define as "the complete integration of traditional and alternative medicines." Regardless of the significance of these three hard-to-ignore factors, the numbers represent a real and measurable trend in how this country views and understands modern medicine.

DR. BARON'S SUPERSTAR HEALTH TIP:

The *new mainstream* is "the complete integration of traditional and alternative medicines."

A "New Mainstream" Awaits

According to the National Center for Complementary and Alternative Medicine (NCCAM) and the National Center for Health Statistics (NCHS), part of the Centers for Disease Control and Prevention, in 1997, Americans spent a staggering $36 - 47 billion dollars on "alternative medicine." These fees represented more than the public paid out-of-pocket for all hospitalizations in 1997 and about half of what was paid for all out-of-pocket physician services. Five billion dollars in out-of-pocket monies was spent on herbal products. This information was released in May 2004 and reflects data that are now over ten years old.[4] The National Health Interview Survey (NHIS) used to compile this data reveals that up to $20 billion dollars was paid out-of-pocket for the services of professional Complimentary and Alternative Medicine (CAM) healthcare providers.

I have called this chapter "The New Mainstream" because that is what my professional athletes and I believe is the future of health care, and the new mainstream is what I am offering you in this very unique book. We have realized that the difference between "mainstream" and "alternative" is purely semantic and that calling anything alternative suggests that it's a substitute for some other, predominant system of service. Health care is not an either/or deal, and what I am proposing should not be considered alternative to anything. Rather, I am asking you to consider taking charge of, and responsibility for, your own well-being in ways that may differ from what you have become accustomed to thinking is "normal." The important thing is not what the particular treatment modality is called but whether it is the right treatment for what ails you and how can you get your hands on it—quickly, safely, and inexpensively.

DR. BARON'S SUPERSTAR HEALTH TIP:

The important thing is not what the particular treatment modality is called but whether it is the right treatment for you and how you can get your hands on it quickly, safely, and inexpensively.

Professional athletes don't have the luxury of choosing one or rejecting another treatment modality; their extreme physical needs require both prevention and a cure—and fast! That is why they demand the best and are provided with the resources to pay for it. So should

---

4

Patricia M. Barnes, E. Powell-Griner, K. McFann, and R. L.. Nahin, *Complementary and Alternative Medicine Use among Adults: United States, 2002*, Advance Data from Vital and Health Statistics, No. 343 (2004), http://nccam.nih.gov/news/report.pdf.

you; and my goal here is to provide you with time-tested and affordable strategies that can make a real difference for you and your well-being. The beauty of the new mainstream medicine I am proposing is that it is ultimately both less costly than traditional medicine and more available. You can participate actively, both in the prevention and the cure; this will enable you to rewire your own fire alarms so that you attend to them sooner. By paying attention to your symptoms earlier, you will hear the alarms less often and retrain yourself to take positive and practical action earlier and more effectively.

DR. BARON'S SUPERSTAR HEALTH TIP:

The beauty of the new mainstream medicine I am proposing is that it is ultimately both less costly than traditional medicine and more available.

So the important question at this point is this: If something could truly help you heal, prevent, and improve your overall health, would you really care who provided it and what he or she called it? I doubt it; the proof is in the results; and that's what I'm offering you in coming chapters as we continue to dismantle the wall that separates "mainstream" from "alternative" and help integrate them into the new mainstream through *Dr. Spencer Baron's Secrets of the Game!*

As we move forward, you'll begin to see what has worked, both through my experiences and through those of my colleagues, with the many professional athletes and other patients we treat on a daily basis. Keep your eyes and ears open as we progress, but more importantly, keep your mind open. Allow yourself to drift past the confines of your general practitioner's office; see past the dog-eared copies of *Highlights* and *Reader's Digest* and move past the walls covered with helpful, healing prints to discover the hidden benefits available through this new mainstream system of identifying and treating your mind and body.

Dr. Baron's Superstar Health Tip:

If something could truly help you heal, prevent, and improve your overall health, would you really care who provided it and what he or she called it?

Chapter 4:

THE ESSENTIAL ATHLETE:

A *Mind* Is a Terrible Thing to Waste

Pressure is something you feel when you don't know what the hell you're doing.
Peyton Manning, Indianapolis Colts

Pressure does one of two things to people. It either crushes you or it turns you into a diamond.
Jason Taylor, 2006 NFL Defensive Player of the Year

Off the Bench and onto the Court: Let's Get Playing!

So now that you understand how we arrived at this point, let's get working on how to put yourself in *peak performance shape.*

First, here's a critical newsflash: If you read and remember *nothing else* in this book, get this—any athlete's ability to succeed is *entirely* driven by his or her will and by his or her intention. It is *not* about the athlete's body. This is as true for Jason Taylor, NFL Miami Dolphins defensive end, as it is for you, me, and everyone we know. Mediocre athletes become superstars because their minds *believe* they are capable of greatness. The most amazing athletes fail, get injured, and lose games not because they are incapable or incompetent, but because of what they *believe*. What you believe your body can do *is* what your body can do.

Nothing else in the rest of this book will be worth any more than the paper it's written on if you do not, clearly and without doubt, understand that your mind drives your body. Once you can control your mind, you can control your body. All of the physical cures, treatments, salves, drugs, home remedies, and other instruments of athletic performance are worthless if your mind does not believe they will work. Conversely, the simplest treatments can work wonders when the mind has powerfully mastered its ability to believe. There is myriad evidence for this in medicine, in sports, and in amazing feats of survival.

For example, the New York Giants' victory in the 2008 Super Bowl could be called an act of sheer determination and will. The Giants were not better players than the New England Patriots, and, in fact, evidence pointed to the contrary, as the Patriots had not lost a single game all season. They were just better able to marshal their powers of intention and determination—both mental processes—to dominate their opponents. It is, thus, quite appropriate that the mantra for New York Giants fans has become: "They wanted it more."

DR. BARON'S SUPERSTAR HEALTH TIP:

**Once you can control your mind,
you can control your body.**

A powerful example of mind over matter can be found during randomized clinical experiments that are used to test the effectiveness of new drugs. In these experiments, some patients are given the actual test drug, while the others are given something like an inert sugar pill, in other words, a placebo. No one is told exactly what he or she is receiving. The drug is said to be effective if it shows a higher success rate at killing the infection than the placebo. What is remarkable about these types of studies is not how they demonstrate success or failure of the drug under study. What is truly remarkable is how often patients receiving the placebo demonstrate results as good as, if not better than, the drug under consideration.

Really think about this. Patients are given a useless pill, and they get better; how strange is that? It's all about the patients' minds *believing* they are being given some powerful new miracle drug that can cure them. And guess what? They get better! Healing is all in the mind, and there are innumerable research studies that support this conclusion.

Hypnosis is another remarkable example of mind over matter. There are many, many studies of the benefits of hypnosis in minimizing pain from medical procedures, headaches, musculoskeletal conditions, irritable bowel syndrome, and fibromyalgia, just to name a few.[5] Hypnosis has also demonstrated particular utility for reducing cancer pain, including bone marrow transplant pain and coping with invasive procedures.[6][7][8] In hypnosis, *absolutely nothing* is done to physically alter the state of the body. This is one of the clearest and most straightforward examples of the mind controlling the body: if you control your mind, you can control your pain.

---

5   H. C. Haanen, H. T. Hoenderdos, L. K. van Romunde, W. C. Hop, C. Mallee, and J. P. Terwiel, "Controlled trial of hypnotherapy in the treatment of refractory fibromyalgia." *Journal of Rheumatology* 18 (1991): 72 –75.

6   G. H. Montgomery, K. N. DuHamel, and W. H. Redd, "A meta-analysis of hypnotically induced analgesia: How effective is hypnosis?" *International Journal of Clinical & Experimental Hypnosis* 48 (2000): 138–53.

7   D. F. Lynch Jr., "Empowering the patient: Hypnosis in the management of cancer, surgical disease and chronic pain," *American Journal of Clinical Hypnosis* 42 (1999): 122–30.

8   E. Ernst, "Complementary therapies in palliative cancer care," *Cancer* 91 (2001): 2181–5; D. L. Handel , "Complementary therapies for cancer patients: What works, what doesn't, and how to know the difference," *Texas Medicine* 97 (2001): 68–73; G. Marchioro, G. Azzarello, F. Viviani, F. Barbato, M. Pavanetto, and F. Rosetti, "Hypnosis in the treatment of anticipatory nausea and vomiting in patients receiving cancer chemotherapy," *Oncology* 59 (2000): 100–104; J. Pattison, "Hypnotherapy: Complementary support in cancer care," *Nursing Standard* 11 (1997): 44–46; D. Renoufe, "Hypnotically induced control of nausea: A preliminary report," *Journal of Psychosomatic Research* 45 (1998): 295–96.

What the Mind Believes, the Body Achieves

The first and most important thing you *must* understand is that your mind, not your body, is running the show. What your mind believes, your body achieves. According to Jimmy Johnson, former head coach of the two-time Super Bowl–winning Dallas Cowboys, "Let the mind control the body, not the body control the mind." If you think you can't do it, guess what? That's right, you can't. Superstar athletes know this, first and foremost. They are *unwilling* to let perceived physical limitations of their bodies stop them.

DR. BARON'S SUPERSTAR HEALTH TIP:

What your mind believes, your body achieves.

Note that I said *perceived*, not real or actual or true or objective. There's a world of difference there. Dr. Jethro Toomer, NFL psychologist, puts it this way: "It's all about perception and how you frame a situation. Did I tell you about the 'Two Sisters'? It is a story of how twin sisters walked into a barn and were confronted with a pile of manure. One sister said, 'Eeww, what a mess!' The other sister said, 'Oh, we have a pony!'"

The same thing goes with your body. One of you will see your poor, tired, out of shape body, and you'll say, "I'll *never* get *this* body into shape." Another will say, "Wow, I am so committed to getting this body into shape; what a great opportunity to show everyone how amazing I am!"

Here's another of Dr. Toomer's examples of the power of perception. He says, "Johnny Bravo is a great cartoon. He's a suave, muscular-looking Elvis, who exhibits exemplary resilience when walking down a city sidewalk as he spots a gorgeous blonde walking her dog in the opposite direction. He stops her to tell her how hot she is and how he would like to get to know her. She hauls off and punches him in the face, knocking him to the floor. He looks into the audience and says, 'See, she can't keep her hands off me.'" It's all in the mind—one man's punch is another man's passion.

In order to achieve peak physical performance, your mind and your body *must* work in concert with one another. There must be a delicate and melodic duet that is always unified and harmonious. It is not unlike a magnificent orchestra that only sounds right when all the instruments are perfectly attuned with one another. The same principle applies to your mind and your body. A mind that cannot control its body is wasted. A body that is not capitalizing on its most powerful tool—its mind—is missing the most important weapon in its entire arsenal. Moreover, if the body is not incorporating all of the nutritional and other methods available, it cannot respond most effectively and efficiently to the mind's commands. In order for the body to operate most efficiently, physical, mental, and nutritional needs must be balanced to create a machine that operates at maximum capacity.

DR. BARON'S SUPERSTAR HEALTH TIP:

In order to achieve peak physical performance, your mind and your body *must* work together.

OK, time for a pop quiz. Question: What is the *single most powerful tool* in the athlete's strategic arsenal?

Answer: HIS MIND!

DR. BARON'S SUPERSTAR HEALTH TIP::

A superstar athlete's single most powerful tool is:
HIS MIND.

I think that everything is possible as long as you put your mind to it and you put the work and time into it. I think your mind really controls everything."
Michael Phelps, winner of eight gold medals, 2008 Summer Olympics

Mental Secrets from Behind the Locker Room Door
Mental Toughness and Resilience

People who have extraordinary athletic competence are masters of what I refer to as *mental toughness* and *resilience*. Consider encountering an unexpected traffic jam on the morning of your big meeting. Some of you will respond by shouting out some choice obscenities to get it out of your system and then move forward with your day as if nothing happened. Mental toughness is this quality of sustaining ideal performance despite whatever life throws at you. In other words, when the going gets tough, the tough get tougher! Mental toughness can be measured by consistent performance, irrespective of time, place, or circumstance. Players who are unfazed by whatever happens around them, good or bad, demonstrate this quality of mental toughness, and they've learned to be mentally tough; it isn't an inherited quality.

Good players use mental toughness throughout their years of training and playing; great players let it use them! What that means is that this attribute has, over time, become so natural and innate that the players never even think about it. They simply *are* mentally tough; there is just no possibility of being any other way.

DR. BARON'S SUPERSTAR HEALTH TIP:

Mental toughness can be measured by consistent performance, irrespective of time, place, or circumstance.

Resilience, on the other hand, describes players who are able to bounce easily and maturely back from adversity. You know that traffic jam I mentioned earlier? Well, resilient drivers will consider it, maybe get upset, call to say they'll be a little late, and then use the valuable extra time to prepare for the meeting or maybe make some important calls they wouldn't otherwise have had time for. They exit the traffic jam feeling productive, empowered, and inspired about the rest of the day. When resilient people face loss, trauma, stress, or injury, they immediately refocus on the future and identify how this event has presented an unexpected opportunity as they move forward. They do not feel defeated or overwhelmed by past events. Resilience is the quality of using adversity as a tool for motivation and inspiration; a resilient player refocuses on the future rather than dwelling on the past.

DR. BARON'S SUPERSTAR HEALTH TIP:

Resilience is using adversity as a tool for motivation and inspiration; a resilient player refocuses on the future rather than dwelling on the past.

The combination of these two characteristics, resilience and mental toughness, enables superstar athletes (and you also, if you so choose) to focus on specific desired results and how best to achieve them. Dr. Toomer suggests that comparing mental toughness and resilience "... is like comparing a 2' x 4' (two by four) piece of wood to a palm tree. One can keep being hit over and over again without a change in their attitude, while the other can sway and bend and resume its position."

What Makes a Great Athlete a Superstar?

As chiropractor for the 1997 World Series-winning Florida Marlins, I treat guys like Kevin Brown, Gary Sheffield, Al Leiter, Bobby Bonilla, Luis Costillo, and Moises Alou all the time. Among winning superstars like these, it is tricky to identify who truly has the winning mind-set. However, as I now enter my fourteenth year treating the Miami Dolphins, who have just experienced their worst season in franchise history, I have had a spectacular opportunity to see who *truly* has mastered mental toughness and resilience. It's when the chips are down that the real superstars emerge.

For example, Jason Taylor's impenetrable ability to play hard, defy injury, and maintain his composure is fast becoming legendary. I don't know what runs though his head on a daily basis, but his actions continue to speak loudly. As of this writing, since 1999, Taylor has started in every single game he has played as a Miami Dolphin—that's 143 games! This alone is a testimonial to tremendous leadership. *Why?* During those 143 games, I've seen Taylor play with fractured bones bearing brand new casts, steel plates and screws in his right arm, and a sprained neck, in addition to sprained fingers, ankles, wrists, and feet. He's played when completely exhausted, with significant mental fatigue, suffering from low back pain, and much, much more. He did this despite playing for a team experiencing one of the worst losing streaks in history; the team's record didn't matter. He still played with 100 percent heart and soul. Now that, my friends, is a superstar.

Some players exhibit great strength and perseverance during the best of times but cannot muster a shred of courage or tenacity when the accolades wane and the winning streak withers. If you really want to see a superstar, go find a losing team and observe who keeps pushing him or herself and his or her team beyond their horizons and the seductive courtship offered by depression and disappointment. Now *there's* your winner! Show me a player who will not accept defeat under any circumstance, and I'll show you a superstar athlete.

DR. BARON'S SUPERSTAR HEALTH TIP:

Show me a player who will not accept defeat under any circumstance, and I'll show you a superstar athlete!

Every major athlete has talent, and every player has the physical ability to be a superstar; otherwise, he or she could not have attracted the attention of that first scout; nor could he or she have been signed by any major team. But the ones who make it are the ones who can control their *minds* whether the team is winning *or* losing. After the season is over, you won't hear much from the athletes who allow negative dramas inside their heads to overcome their drive and motivation. Remember Bobbie Fisher, the supreme grandmaster who put the exceedingly mental sport of chess on the map and into our national consciousness? (Now, when you think about it, who had ever heard of chess—much less considered it a *sport*—before or, for that matter, even after Bobby Fisher?) After being the first American to win the World Chess Championships in 1972, his anti-American and anti-Semitic beliefs fueled his rapid fall from grace. His once escalating base of popular support gave way to consensus that his negative thoughts and paranoid delusions made him unworthy of being hailed as one of the greatest thinkers of the century.

So, now that we're clear how essential the mind is to generating winning performance, let's look at some of the specific tips and techniques that superstar athletes keep locked in their mental treasure chest of secrets to help them overcome odds and become superstars. In chapter 5, I'll give you some great tips and techniques for exploiting your mind in service of your body.

Remember, your mind is either your greatest asset or your strongest opponent; use it wisely!

Chapter 5:

THE ESSENTIAL ATHLETE:

Mental Secrets of the Superstar Athletes

Now that you know your mind is either your greatest ally or your most determined foe, you get to choose how you want to use it. As you read this chapter, you'll see some great strategies for how you can use your mind to your greatest advantage and how superstar athletes use these same methods to control their own wandering minds. My intention is to give you clear explanations and examples that will help you understand what I'm talking about, as well as illustrations directly from the mouths of amazing athletes who agreed to share their secrets with me for this book.

Secret of the Mind #1:
Outwit Your Ineffective Thinking

Ineffective thinking can drain your mental and your physical resources. When your mind says you feel sick, you feel sick. When your mind says you are capable, you feel capable. Ineffective thinking is at the source of many an athlete's demise.

According to Dr. Kevin Elko, renowned sports psychologist and motivational speaker, five key sources of ineffective thinking bring athletes down, and overcoming these is critical to speeding healing and improving performance. In his words, forms of ineffective thinking such as:

> Exaggeration (I will never play again), overgeneralization (my decision on that first play cost us the season), invalidated assumptions (the coach hates me because he didn't say hello today), illogic [conclusions] (what is the use anyway), and faulty deductions (I do not have to rehabilitate, I will be fine) ... will sabotage rehabilitation as well as playoff performances.[9]

Each of these irrational beliefs completely demoralizes an athlete. An athlete who indulges in this line of thinking distorts reality despite his subjective belief in his own rationality. When an athlete uses extreme words like "awful," "terrible," or "horrible" to describe her performance, she allows her mind to lead her body into debilitating despair. Sometimes, simply changing the words that describe the event can significantly affect the athlete's ability to reframe and recover from a disappointing incident. An attentive coach might suggest changing "hate" to "dislike" (my mom's personal favorite) or "problems" to "challenges." The coach hopes to stimulate inspiration rather than perspiration!. Consider what happens when you shift "This is killing me" to "This hurts really badly" and then to "This hurts." Softening the words can minimize negative and enhance positive impacts. Get the point? It's all in your vocabulary!

---

9   F. H. Fu, F. H. and D. A. Stone. 2001. Sports Injuries: *Mechanisms, Prevention, Treatment*. Philadelphia, PA: Lippincott Williams & Wilkins.

Secret of the Mind #2:
Find Your Most Powerful Leaders

Good leadership is essential to success. Great leadership is indispensable to masterful teamwork and award-winning performance. I have watched the styles of six different Miami Dolphins' head coaches, beginning with Don Shula, who landed in the 1997 Pro Football Hall of Fame and was known as "the winningest head coach in professional football history."[10] I watched Jimmy Johnson, who previously led the Dallas Cowboys to two Super Bowl victories, all the way through to Cam Cameron and now his replacement, Tony Sparano. Each coach was confident that he could ultimately lead the Dolphins to victory. Each was a powerful strategic coach in his own right but missed the elusive Super Bowl victory (with the exception of Coach Shula). In fact, in 2007, the Dolphins experienced their worst record in franchise history.

So what happens when leaders cannot effectively lead their athletes?

One of the most important aspects of powerful athletic leadership is strong personal presence. It's similar to the charismatic quality a great actor uses to make you believe in her character. It's about demonstrating unshakeable power and influence, whether it's genuine or not. Some might term it, "fake it till you make it," or more aptly in this case, "never let 'em see you sweat!" No matter what, a great leader never lets the people around him witness uncertainty or indecision when coaching the team, no matter what is going on inside.

I remember an airline trip I once took from Fort Lauderdale, Florida, to New York City when the weather was pretty dicey. After an hour in the air and some minor turbulence, I headed for my "seventh-inning stretch." As I exited the restroom, the turbulence suddenly hit about a 7 on the Richter scale. Despite my initial anxiety, I managed to stay calm while I did a quick mental check to assure myself that everyone was okay.

The plane leveled, and then—WHAM!—another jolt of turbulence

---

10   http://www.profootballhof.com/history/decades/1990s/don_shula.jsp ,
Official Site of the Pro Football Hall of Fame

shook the plane like Ryan Newman's spectacular crash on lap 53 at the 2003 Daytona 500 (OK, so maybe that's a *little* exaggerated). Again, I was fine, *until* I saw the panic-stricken faces of two different flight attendants; this was not good! My mind began to send warning signals throughout my body, as my calm exterior quickly deteriorated into unnerving fear. "Ohmygosh," I thought, "if *the experts* are upset, then I better get with the program here!"

I saw how my mind was beginning to send physical symptoms of panic into my impressionable body (palms sweating, heart racing, legs shaking), and I realized that I'd better redirect my mind to believe that we'd be just fine, or I'd lose it. As I quieted and took control of my mind, my fear gradually transformed back to calm. My point is this: a leader has a responsibility to stay composed in spite of any real or imagined breakdown because others will naturally follow her lead. If the flight attendants had remained calm, I would naturally have followed their lead. The tip is this: pick your leaders carefully; they have tremendous influence over your performance, whether you realize it or not.

Secret of the Mind #3:
Resist "Mind Rot"

Here's how to prevent what I call "mind rot"—you know, that insidious disease that infects your brain and makes it spew negativity all around you like nuclear fallout.

There are some basic principles that all infections share: first, if left unattended, they will increase in size; and, second, they will contaminate everything they touch. Infection is all around us; and, thanks to Louis Pasteur, everyone knows that if an open wound is exposed to germs, bacteria, viruses, and other bugs, it becomes infected. Preventing this process requires two basic strategies: (1) keep out the contaminants and (2) strengthen your immune system.

Your mind operates in precisely the *same* way. When negative or "infectious" thoughts intrude, they will germinate and take over all the uninfected areas. To avoid contamination, you *must*: (1) avoid negative people whose intention, consciously or not, is to drag you down with them (you know how misery just *loves* company) and (2) strengthen your mindset as you would your immune system—give it the tools to fight back and resist infection.

So, you ask, how do I do that?

Well, rather than take it from me, here's what runs through the minds of "super slugs" just before they become superheroes. This is what superstar athletes do to overcome that potentially overwhelming temptation to slip into self-defeating mental contamination.

> *Following a negative thought, my mind goes blank; then I think of something ...an extremely inspiring time with grandma, wife or son. As the bad stuff tunes out, I feel a sudden moment of intense energy to call out plays in the huddle and go back to winning.*
>
> **Ray Philyaw**, quarterback, Cleveland Gladiators, Arena Football League

---

Secret of the Mind #4:
The Drills Are Alive ... with the Sound of Music

What is it about the sound of music that stirs the soul and tickles the fancy of athletic prowess? No matter what the genre—classical, jazz, hip-hop, rock, or reggae—musical stimulation can fuel incredible feats of mind over matter vis-à-vis athletic performance and temporary pain relief. A recent study even showed that rock music improved optimism and reduced pessimism among university-level psychology and music students.[11] (How about that, parents? It's actually good for them.)

Music can have various effects, and you want to use just the right type for the occasion. Your music should set just the right mood but also conserve your energy for that ultimate climax at the end (yes, the not-so-subtle analogy here *is* intentional). You see, while music can effectively generate adrenaline right before a competition, athletes

---

11   V. N. Stratton, "Daily Music Listening Habits in College Students: Related Moods and Activities." *Psychology and Education: An Interdisciplinary Journal* 40 (2003): 1–11, news release, Penn State University.

must be careful not to bring on too much too soon or they may lose their vital *energy* before the big moment arrives. Because adrenaline is a short-acting hormone, it can dwindle just when it is required most because your body does not store and then release it as necessary. When you are performing, so many chemicals cascade through your veins to feed your muscles and brain that you want to make sure you maintain your competitive edge as long and as consistently as possible. The right music can help you do this.

Here are some examples: Let's say that you are preparing for a competitive event that requires higher cognition— a spelling bee or a chess match—or you're rigorously studying the playbook for the big soccer, basketball, or hockey game. In that case, Mozart is your man (or boy, since he began composing at the ripe old age of four), as you want to improve memory and problem solving. Classical music, particularly Mozart's sonatas, has been found to enhance brain function consistent with what psychologists refer to as spatial-temporal reasoning. This is the type of logic that people who are good at things like architecture, engineering, science, mathematics, art, and games use.[12]

When studying, you should listen to music that doesn't have words, which will distract your brain and clog your recall patterns. For memory retention, the harpsichord is your instrument. This instrument naturally induces and relaxes alpha-brainwave activity, which is consistent with higher-level learning. (Following this section, is a list of brainwave inducing musical pieces that I would listen to during the writing of this book.)[13]

---

12   J. Renz and B. Nebel, "Qualitative Spatial Reasoning using Constraint Calculi" in: M. Aiello, I. Pratt-Hartmann, J. van Benthem (eds.), *Handbook of Spatial Logics*, Kluwer, Springer Netherlands, 2007, pages 161-215.
13   Dr. Baron's music for memory:
   Vivaldi
   Largo from "Winter" from The Four Seasons
   Largo from Concerto in D Major for Guitar and Strings
   Largo from Concerto in C Major for Mandolin, Strings, and Harpsichord
   Telemann
   Largo from Double Fantasia in G Major for Harpsichord
   Bach, J. S.
   Largo from Harpsichord Concert in F Minor, BWV 1056
   Air for the G String
   Largo from Harpsichord Concerto in C. Major BWV 975

Secret of the Mind #5:
Very Superstitious Writings on the Wall

I have got this obsessive compulsive disorder where I have to have everything in a straight line, or everything has to be in pairs.
David Beckham, Los Angeles Galaxy, Major League Soccer

"When you believe in things that you don't understand, then you suffer." Love the song, but I'm not sure Stevie Wonder got it quite right when it comes to sports; professional athletes are *nuts* about routine and control, even if they can't explain *why* they do what they do. Ever see a baseball pitcher touch his cap the same way before every pitch or a football player remove his mouthpiece a certain way after every play? How about the way a basketball player laces his sneakers? And then there's the baseball coach who wears the same underwear every day during playoffs (don't you just wish I could tell you who *that* is?!) But do these weird routines really work?

"No!" the pragmatist in you says, "don't be ridiculous!"

Now, I'm no psychologist, but there is something to the way our routines make us feel secure and thus help us perform better. You can even see this with little babies and small children; when their lives are organized into predictable and stable routines, they are calmer and more relaxed. The comfort and security of knowing what will come next helps them feel in control in an otherwise overwhelming and chaotic world.

As adults, we are not so different, and this same basic principle is at work with superstar athletes. Each time the coach instructs the athlete to lean forward to perfect his vault off the springboard, or to trap the soccer ball with her left foot, his or her brain is being conditioned to repeat certain concepts. Little by little, the athlete begins to "believe in things that [he or she doesn't] understand," as suggested by the illustrious Stevie Wonder. Truth to tell, we're not that different from poor Pavlov's dog, which was conditioned to expect food every time a bell rang. Eventually, that poor dog began to salivate at the mere ringing of a bell in anticipation of his savory morsels, even if none appeared.

Coaches and athletic trainers use the same conditioning principle to train superstar athletes.

Remember how I used to wrestle when I was a teen? Well, every time I prepared to execute my "hotshot" fireman's carry wrestling maneuver, my body and mind were busily reviewing thousands of bits of information as I angled for the takedown. I instantaneously analyzed the smell in the air, the music in the background, the colors in my peripheral vision, and the fabric on my skin, as I mapped my "perfect plan." Before I knew it, all of the significant and insignificant stimuli coalesced to have me salivating when the bell rang. Yeah, we're all just like Pavlov's dog; our conditioning determines what we anticipate and, thus, how we respond.

So, you tell me—what the heck does always wearing your college shorts underneath your NBA uniform have to do with winning a playoff game, *superstar Michael Jordan*? Carlos Delgado of the New York Mets said in a personal interview: "There is a baseball joke that says the only superstition is that, after you hit the ball, you must touch every base." (Yes, that would make for a homerun.)

The bottom line is simple. If you fundamentally believe that something is going to work for you every time, then as long as it's safe and does not harm anyone else, power to you! So, if you want to sleep with your baseball bat the night before a big game, then go right ahead. Just make sure your spouse is with the program, or the resulting bedroom chill might undercut the thrill of your victory!

Secret of the Mind #6:
Get Psyched!

Remember in chapter 1 when I explained all about the mind/body connection and how it developed? Well, despite considerable evidence to the contrary, many athletes continue to operate on the antiquated assumption that the mind and body can indeed be separated. Even professional athletes, who masterfully blend the ideals of Eastern and Western medicine while caring for their bodies, may forget that essential mind/body connection at crucial moments.

When training your mind to support your athletic performance, you might have had one of several experiences: You may never have competed before and have no experience of winning or losing. Alternatively, you may have competed before and won; or you may have competed before and lost. Each of these scenarios has powerfully created your relationship to competition and athletic achievement.

However, none of these experiences makes much difference in predicting the likelihood that you will win or lose the next time. What *does* make a difference, however, is what your mind tells you and how carefully you monitor your thoughts. No matter how perfectly primed your body may be, your negative thoughts may sabotage your best efforts at success.

What works is to visualize every step of your success and then act accordingly. It's not good enough to just create an image of crossing the finish line or sinking the winning jump shot or whatever it may be for you. Rather, you must precisely visualize *every single detail* necessary to accomplish your desired result. You must vividly mentally experience, not just think about, the *whole* race, from start to finish. At the same time, closely watch your favorite top athlete. Study his or her actions and then seize them as your own. Remember, the devil is in the details, and limiting yourself to the "big picture" will defeat your ambition.

"So," you say, "what about when I keep losing, and I just can't seem to get it right?"

"Get over it," I say.

That is, connect to the feeling and sensation of winning, and recondition your mind to visualize you as a winner who is capable of amazing victories. Connect with extraordinary experiences you've had, such as the day you held your child for the first time or your wedding day (hopefully this was a good experience!) or the day you won a spelling bee or were elected to a coveted position. Mentally revert to these moments, as you build confidence in your capacity and then transpose it onto the current experience you are attempting to have. Tell yourself things like, "If I can give birth, I can certainly win *this* race." Or, say, "I got that job over the 300 fabulous people who also applied; *of course* I can beat a mere 20 of the best divers in this championship." Piece o' cake! Sounds trite, I know, but it really works.

Try it and see what happens. Then, if you don't notice a difference, let me know, and we'll see what went wrong.

Secret of the Mind #7:
Do It or Die Trying!

OK, here's the best way I can explain this one. At the moment of each of my sons' births (I have two), I knew beyond the shadow of a doubt and without a moment's hesitation that I would take a bullet to prevent *anything* or *anyone* from harming them. That's how clear I was about what mattered most to me at that moment.

Our brave men and women in military service experience the same irrefutable dedication; these are men and women who put their lives on the line every second of every day in service of their country. For others, the driving force an ideal; Mahatma Gandhi, Martin Luther King, and John F. Kennedy are all examples of people whose principles gave meaning and direction to their lives. This is the kind of drive and focus that you must bring to your health and well-being and, in turn, your athletic performance.

I had an experience of this sort quite recently. In fact, it was while I was writing this book. Every year in February, I participate in a half marathon in Fort Lauderdale that I use to test my athletic ability and see how I have improved over the past year. But this year, I *really* did not want to run. I was at the tail end of a painful divorce, I was struggling financially, my beloved father was quickly dying from pancreatic cancer, and a significant injury to my leg all left me clear that this was *not* the year to test my physical ability. It would simply be an exercise in self-sabotage.

Despite all my considerations and my circumstances, I entered the race. My training was going poorly, as I had barely been able to complete a five-mile run for the past two weeks. For me, that was really pathetic. Then I said, "The hell with it." I could worry and struggle and suffer over all the miserable moments in my life, or I could just get over it. As I considered my father lying there in pain feeling his life ebb slowly away, all of my issues seemed to pale in comparison. So, I just picked myself up and I ran.

And I ran.

And I ran.

I never felt so much emotional and physical pain during a competition. But once I realized that all of this "stuff" going on in my life was just "stuff" and that I could let it get in my way or not, I ran with abandon toward the finish line, where my two magnificent sons were waiting. My agony slowly transformed into joy, and I finished the race not a minute slower than the last year, holding my older son's hand as I completed the final 20 yards. It was truly one of the most memorable moments of my life; I wouldn't trade one minute of it for anything.

Anything can be a "do or die" in your mind; you get to make the final call. What will it take for you to find the inner strength to overcome an obstacle?

So what will you take a stand for and believe with every cell in your body? Imagine what you could do with that kind of unstoppable energy. That's the kind of commitment that superstar athletes must put into each and every game. By bringing that perseverance and dedication to your own efforts, you can achieve unimaginable results.

You have to believe in yourself when no one else does—
that makes you a winner right there.
Venus Williams, Woman's Professional Tennis

All my life I've had to fight. It's just another fight I'm going to have to
learn how to win, that's all.
Serena Williams, Woman's Professional Tennis

Secret of the Mind #8:
Gotta Get Your "Want to" Up!

You can't control your level of talent, but you can control your level of effort.
Thomas Blake, Pro tennis player, James Blake's father[14]

---

14   J. Blake, *Breaking Back*, (New York: Harper Collins Publishers, 2007), 154.

How often do you talk yourself *out* of doing things? You planned to go for a run, play with the kids, practice your golf swing, or ride your bike, and then it just seemed like too ... much ... work. Maybe finishing the chapter in a good book detained you or sleeping in or watching the last contestant get booted out on *American Idol.* (You know, the *really* important stuff!)

Now here's the thing: *How you do anything is how you do everything!* It's never *just* this game, *just* this moment, or *just* this incident.

Whether you can see it or not, you always bring the same you—with all your excuses, strategies, conditions, and whatever else—into every aspect of your life, on the court and off. You are the same you at work, with your family, and with your body. We all have our individual strategies for getting motivated and accomplishing tasks. For me, I have learned that I need a coach who snaps at my butt like a nasty crocodile to hold me accountable for accomplishing what I say I will accomplish. Now, just for the record, let me assure you I am extremely self-motivated; I'm up at 4:30 a.m. every day, at the gym by 5:30 a.m., and working by 7:00 a.m. For me, getting the miserable task of weight training done means I better do it first thing or it ain't gonna happen. I know that, left to my own devices, a lot of things won't happen that I am committed to, unless I set up some external accountability to "get my want to up" about a lot of things. So, I hire a fabulous life coach who helps me set goals and then figure out how to accomplish them as efficiently and effectively as possible.

This might not be the most effective strategy for you. That's fine. Your job is to find out what gets you going and then go do it! Figuring out your own unique code for getting the job done is as good as gold. Maybe you need a training partner, a coach, a mentor, someone to nurture you, or someone to kick your butt. Maybe it's just tracking your times and setting personal goals for yourself each week. Whatever it is, set it up and use it.

I don't play for records. I have pride! I go out there and respect the game and myself. I will not embarrass myself or my team.
Carlos Delgado, New York Mets, Major League Baseball

Secret of the Mind #9:
Get Razzled and Bedazzled!

I don't want to be the next Michael Jordan, I only want to be Kobe Bryant.
Kobe Bryant, Los Angeles Lakers, National Basketball Association

Ever wonder what LeBron James thinks as he floats through the air or what Kobe Bryant thinks as he hits his amazing three-pointers? What do you think motivates *them*? What inspires *them*? *How* do they make themselves *do* that?! In other words, what do you think excites LeBron James or Kobe Bryant? Even as you watch, awestruck by some flawless act of sheer physical brilliance that seems inconceivable, do you ever consider what gives *them* goose bumps and makes the hair on *their* arms stand on end?

Getting inspired is one of the most important aspects of superior athletic performance and staying healthy. It starts when you are a small child and continues to shake, rattle, and roll you as you move through your life. No one ever got to be the best at anything without first being inspired by something or someone. That's what led a progression of subsequent runners to beat Roger Bannister's record-breaking four-minute mile in 1954. And, once you've been there, you can never go back.

Many people admire John F. Kennedy and Martin Luther King, as do I. Why? Because their words and actions inspire and motivate me to be a better person. As master communicators, each managed to convey his own deep sense of belief, power, and commitment to his ideals. Look at Stephen Hawking, a theoretical physicist, known for quantum gravity, black holes, and theoretical cosmology—and a quadriplegic, paralyzed by ALS (Amyotrophic Lateral Sclerosis). He has managed to achieve more in one lifetime than most us could do in ten. He says:

I am quite often asked: How do you feel about having ALS? The answer is, not a lot. I try to lead as normal a life as possible, and not think about my condition, or regret the things it prevents me from doing, which are not that many.[15]

---

15   Stephen Hawking, "Disability" *www.hawking.org.uk*, http://www.hawking.org.uk/disable/dindex.html.

I believe that you and I are not too different when we look deep inside ourselves at what we really want (whether or not we believe we are capable of it). Ultimately, I believe we all want to be able to make that kind of a difference in the world and inspire others to do the same.

Maybe someone inspires you in a glance or even in a televised encounter that leaves you speechless. That's what happened to me when I saw actress Glenn Close on *LIVE with Regis and Kelly* one Friday morning. Something clicked the minute I saw her, and I fell in love (no, I am not a stalker, and she remains blissfully unaware of my infatuation). It was not her looks, as she's not "beautiful," but rather how she appeared so exquisitely at ease in her own skin. With remarkable poise and grace, she seemed to float onstage and answer questions with such comfort, dignity, and style, as if there was nothing to prove and no one to prove it to. "That," I thought, "is what *I* want!"

Closer to home, I remain moved and touched by my own father (who tragically went from diagnosis to death from pancreatic cancer as I struggled with writing chapters 4 and 5 of this book). Everyone around him, including, and perhaps most especially, me, admired his remarkable integrity, punctuality, intelligence, humor, and congeniality. Now, more than ever, I am committed to emulating these qualities, as I reflect on and honor his life and the gifts he left me.

Tell me, who inspires you? Who do you admire and have always wished to be like? It might be someone you know well, like a family member, friend, or work colleague, or someone you've never met who inspires you from afar. There may be more than one person you admire.

Here's why it's so important to identify those you admire—you tend to take on the qualities of people you hang around with or look up to. Since these folks can be either good or bad influences, why not choose people who cause you to be a better, rather than a worse, version of yourself? If you hang around with people you think know more or who have skills and attributes you'd like for yourself, then, over time, you tend to acquire those qualities, too. It's virtually impossible not to.

So, what's amazing to the amazing? Who do the athletes at the top of their game admire most?

I admire my father's ability to work hard, stay focused, and treat people with respect—the key to success is building healthy relationships.
Chad Pennington, Miami Dolphins quarterback,
National Football League

Secret of the Mind #10:
Enter the "Mentor Center."

Your mentor guides, teaches, and sets an example for you. She supports you in accomplishing your own goals and gives you concrete ways to do so. You choose her because you trust her expertise, so you don't have to "reinvent the wheel," or figure out how to consistently swing a golf club like Tiger Woods or maneuver a race car like Jeff Gordon. Mentorship is part teaching and part leading by example. In her role as your teacher, your mentor may videotape your swing and compare it your favorite pro on a split screen monitor; she helps you get clear on what you're aiming for and then motivates you to achieve it. As an example, your mentor may be an exceptional golfer, who has dedicated her life to perfecting her sport and passing that knowledge on to others.

Your mentor may come in many shapes and sizes and may show up when you least expect him. I have had several mentors, most recently a petite, highly-motivated, spiritually-driven powerhouse of a human: my life coach, Nancy Powers. Now, I've had big, hulking training partners in the gym, brilliant business and financial consultants, accountants, and whiz-kid associate doctors in the office. You name it; I've had a consultant or a coach for it. My former wife and I even had a birthing coach during the delivery of our first son. But never, ever have I had a miniature Tony Robbins slice and dice my world like Nancy does. She gets down to the core of what I do and why I do it! She "gets" me at the deepest level … and then goes in for the one-two punch. She helps me find my own self-expression, acknowledges my attributes, and empowers me to find my own answers. To me, she is an extraordinary "princess of power" and an extraordinary mentor.

Mom is my mentor—she always believed in me.

Coach Mike Wilpolt,
2007 Coach of the Year,
Arena Football League

Secret of the Mind #11:
Be Your Own Best Inspiration

Here's the bottom line. You can admire people all day long for what they have accomplished against the odds, but ultimately none of that really matters. What matters is what *you've* been through and how it has affected you. During my 23 years as a practicing chiropractor, I am never more humbled than when I hear what my patients have experienced and how they have coped. Maybe you need to be amazed at what *you* have done instead of minimizing your own accomplishments and mumbling under your breath that, well, "Anyone could have done that." Maybe someone else could have done what you did, but maybe not.

Maybe *you* should be the superstar of your own life.

Take an inventory of your victories. Look into your own life and see where you've succeeded against the odds. If you can't find it, ask your friends, ask your family, ask your teachers, ask *anybody*! Have you ever heard the expression "taking many years to become an overnight success?" The road paved with your own blood, sweat, and tears is the one that has brought you to where you now stand or has enabled you to see where you want to be. Here's the thing: we are usually the last ones to recognize and accept our own greatness. And, quite frankly, if you are not your own biggest champion, why ever would you expect anyone else to be?

If you were watching you, what would excite you? Perhaps it was something that no one knows about; perhaps the people around you, such as, your kids, parents, family, friends, peers, etc. should know, perhaps not—that's your call. Maybe your best accomplishment is something everyone knows about, but your friends and family only seen the end result; no one really knows all the work it took to get there.

Here's what some of the greats say about their own lives and experiences.

> *I am proud of my refusal to fail. So many people want to succeed, but are afraid to fail. They never let themselves be great. The fear of what might happen, negatively, is too much for them to do the things they really want to do to accomplish what they want to accomplish. Likewise, I would hope I inspire people for my willingness to try things outside of my realm and comfort zone.*
> **Jason Taylor**, Miami Dolphins, National Football League

Secret of the Mind #12:
Be a Magnet for Good Advice

Everyone has something to tell you. You can get advice from the newspaper, the television, your friends, your mother(!), *Cosmopolitan* magazine, *Men's Health* magazine, Dear Abby, Ann Landers, Miss Manners, Dr. Phil, Martha Stewart, Maury Povich, *Doonesbury*, Charlie Brown … aaiiieee! Make it stop! There's so much coming at you that sometimes it may seem like everyone knows what's best for you but you.

But get this. Some of this is good advice.

Being able to separate "the wheat from the chaff" may be one of your best assets. Do you realize that one simple piece of good advice might alter the course of your *whole life*? I got my life-altering piece of advice one day, many years ago, during a routine workout at my local gym. In the middle of some conversation I don't quite remember, with some guy I don't quite remember, he advised me that, "Your job should be something that would allow you to be happy *every* day." I thought about it for some time and then realized that what would truly make me happy would be to: (1) help support people in managing their own health and well-being, (2) be my own boss, (3) use my creativity, and (4) do something involving sports. As a result, here I am, living my own version of the dream. For me, this path has enabled me to do what

1970s rock and roller Ted Nugent once expressed in a radio interview. "I work hard to earn my pay, lucky for me, my work is play."

It's a scary thought, isn't it? If you are reading this book, you are looking for some good advice right here, and this is an opportunity for you to practice what I am suggesting. Not everything here will be right for you, but so what?

Take what works and leave the rest. Trust your own instinct on this and consider that everything in this book is only a suggestion. I know it all works, but only you know what works best for you. If one bit of advice in this book helps you beyond your expectations, then you have done what all professional athletes have done at one time or another in their lives. They have learned to discern what best suits them and to discard the rest. You can, too, and here are some hints for helping you do that.

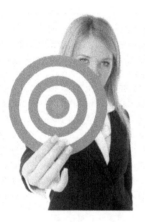

Step 1: Be Intentional – Your thoughts will attract and produce the life experiences that you desire most. It's like taking a trip and using a road map; if you don't know where you're going, then the map is irrelevant, and any road will take you there; but you just might wind up *nowhere*! If you create your goals and put them at the center of your awareness, it's like putting them in the center of the bull's-eye in target practice. You must focus on the center, the thing you want the most. For sharp shooters or archers, this is a piece of cake. For most of us, it may be a bit harder to believe that our thoughts have this kind of power. So get a target for your wall. Write your personal goals right in the center and then use this to focus on your life's desires right there in the center of the target.

Step 2: Start Small and Watch the Change Happen. Try this experiment. Think about buying a yellow car. Then, as you're driving, see how many yellow cars suddenly appear on the road. Suddenly, it seems like there are an awful lot of yellow cars out there, right? It's the same with your goals. Once you focus on them, they start to materialize, as if from nowhere. Look into your life and see where you have made things happen. Allow those life experiences to override your doubts. Once you achieve some easy milestones, aim for the bigger ones. Once you hit the black and the white target zones (that is, you achieve some portion of your goal, or you achieve your goal but not quite the way you 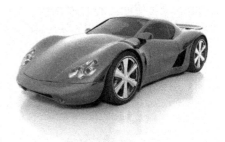 anticipated), then step it up to the red and the blue zones of the target. Now you are building enough confidence to hit the yellow center.

Step 3: Be Aware – Start paying attention as good advice seems to find you. As you start getting clear on your goals, you'll automatically become good at making choices and decisions that are consistent with these goals. At the same time, you'll begin to notice how good advice seems to find you; you don't even have to go looking for it.

The point is this: If you know what you want to achieve and you are clear about your own intention, then the counsel, the friendship, the motivation—the right pieces of your achievement puzzle—show up, and you automatically begin to discard the stuff that isn't for you. Seeking out the advice and support you need to achieve your goals becomes habitual as you learn to trust your own instinct and train your mind to consciously filter information.

The bottom line is this: Advice is truly what you make of it.

Summary

Recall the pop quiz I gave you at the beginning of this section, where I asked what was the most important tool an athlete possessed. You said, HIS MIND! Now we've learned a bit more about how to make the most of what your mind has to offer you. We've learned in this chapter that the mind is central to achieving peak performance and keeping your body healthy and injury free. Controlling your mind is ultimately as important, if not more so, than controlling your body.

Here's a recap of my Secret's of the Mind:

Secret of the Mind #1: Outwit Your Ineffective Thinking. Watch your language, be careful how you express yourself, and try not to use extremes when you evaluate your own performance.

Secret of the Mind #2: Find Your Most Powerful Leaders. Locate and align yourself with great leadership.

Secret of the Mind #3: Resist "Mind Rot." Dominate your negative thoughts before they dominate you.

Secret of the Mind #4: The Drills Are Alive ... with the Sound of Music. Use music to motivate, inspire, and energize you.

Secret of the Mind #5: Very Superstitious Writings on the Wall .... Use any belief or superstition if it helps you, while not hurting or offending anyone else.

Secret of the Mind #6: Get Psyched! Use positive past experiences to help build and strengthen your commitment to athletic achievement.

Secret of the Mind #7: Do It or Die Trying! Be clear on what matters to you and use that as inspiration and motivation.

Secret of the Mind #8: Gotta Get Your "Want to" Up! Find your best strategies to motivate and hold yourself accountable.

Secret of the Mind #9: Get Razzled and Bedazzled!
Identify what inspires you and use it—a lot!

Secret of the Mind #10: Enter the "Mentor Center."
Find a terrific mentor you respect and let her or him educate and lead you.

Secret of the Mind #11: Be Your Own Best Inspiration.
Be inspired by your own accomplishments and make sure you are your own best cheerleader.

Secret of the Mind #12: Be a Magnet for Good Advice. Clarify your goals and then search out and let good advice find you.

I would suggest typing these out and putting them somewhere so that you can be reminded of them all the time. Better yet, go to my website at www.DrSpencerBaron.com to get your free copy of all the secrets in this book in an attractive and user-friendly form. The printout makes not using the secrets virtually impossible. And how about this for some incentive: enter the code ENERGY, and I'll give you three additional secrets not included in the book!

Now, let's move on to the next critical factor in getting your body in peak performance shape: how to use nutrition to strengthen, energize, and heal your body!

Chapter 6

THE ESSENTIAL ATHLETE:

Understanding Diet and Ultimate Liquid Nutritional Strategies

"Health" is a multifaceted and multilayered concept. As I discussed in the last section, you are not a one-dimensional being but, rather, for optimal health, you must honor your mental, nutritional, and physical needs. Each of these is essential to an overall state of health or what is perhaps better referred to as "well-being." We've already covered mental conditioning in chapters 4 and 5. Now, let's focus on some tried and true nutritional strategies that keep superstar athletes performing at their best and that can considerably improve your own energy, performance, and results. The recommendations in this chapter come from a variety of sources, ranging from highly paid doctors to athletic trainers and coaches to individual superstar to Grandma's home remedies.

... lifting weights four times a week, snacking on fresh fruit and vegetables, and exploring cycling and running trails at every NASCAR tour stop.

Carl Edwards, NASCAR

Here's a really important hint: *It doesn't have to cost a lot for it to work.* In fact, it doesn't have to cost at all; it just has to work! As we proceed, I'll give you clear, easy-to-understand-and-apply nutritional strategies for keeping your body in top form.

One of the most important things you can do for your body is to keep it properly hydrated. In this chapter, we'll concentrate on how to get and properly use all the liquids you need for optimal performance. Remember, your body is made up of about 60 percent water, so it's one of the most essential elements for keeping your body strong, healthy, and fit. I'll begin by giving you a brief overview of the role of proper diet in optimal health, and then I'll sail right into ideal hydration secrets.

Dr. Baron's Superstar Health Tip:

Your body is made up of about 60 percent water, so water is one of the most essential elements for keeping your body strong, healthy, and fit.

The Role of Nutrition in Physical Well-Being

Early on, medical doctors believed that food had little to do with well-being, and there was little or no knowledge about the vital role of vitamins in a balanced diet or in overall physical health. Believe it or not, in the 1960s, the American Medical Association even used to advocate cigarette smoking! Can you even *imagine* getting away with that now?

Once the essential importance of vitamins and minerals in the diet was clearly established, popular belief held that we get all the nutrients we need from the food we eat and that additional supplements were unnecessary. This *would* be true if indeed we actually ate the healthy, nutritious, and balanced diets we are supposed to. But with a fast, easy, and cheap McDonald's, Burger King, Taco Bell, Wendy's, Kentucky Fried Chicken, and such on every corner, the temptation to slide into blissful fast-food euphoria can be irresistible. Moreover, many fast-food chains now claim that their food is actually healthy and nutritious, and devious advertising helps assuage our guilt and suck us right in, like a tearful Hallmark commercial promising our problems will be solved by delivering one happy, sappy card. Most of us have long since forgotten what's considered "healthy" eating, as good habits have been lost in the demands of a life overwhelmed with getting the kids to school, working, caring for aging parents, soccer practice, ballet recitals, baseball games, homework, and cocktails with friends; who has time to eat well?

DR. BARON'S SUPERSTAR HEALTH TIP:

Most of us have long since forgotten what's considered "healthy" eating.

The result is that the traditional diet of "three square meals" has given way to easier, faster, and chemically adulterated foods that have become the implicit industry standard. Big food-manufacturing companies and fast-food restaurants have added many unnecessary chemicals to preserve flavor, enhance color, and improve taste, while the devastating impact on our bodies has gone unnoticed. Get this: our bodies have become so chemically well preserved that even the folks who run our burial grounds have expressed concern that our bodies are *decaying* at measurably slower rates today than 100 years ago!

For heaven's sake, we're not even decomposing properly.

The old saying, "You are what you eat," has now been transformed into "You are what you assimilate." This "new" paradigm suggests that one of two things may have occurred: (1) we may be eating nutritionally rich food but have become unable to absorb its benefits properly due to years of digestive system neglect, or (2) the food itself no longer provides the right combination of nutrients to support our now chemically and biologically altered bodies.

DR. BARON'S SUPERSTAR HEALTH TIP:

It's no longer, "You are what you eat." It's now, "You are what you assimilate."

For example, we have all been raised on the unshakable belief that milk is a great source of calcium and other vitamins; the dairy industry has fashioned "Got Milk?" into a household phrase. Yet, why then are we the only animals encouraged to drink this stuff into and through adulthood? Have you ever heard of being lactose intolerant? This is when ingesting milk or any dairy product causes stomach pain, bloating, gas, or diarrhea. This is because, while milk may be nutritious (and a heck of a lot better than soda), many adults stop producing the digestive enzymes (called lactase) that enable us to break down and digest milk beyond childhood. Some of us remain so determined to scoop up that ice cream and chow down that cheese, that we'd rather take a pill than deal with the reality that our bodies are not designed to ingest this food. Remember that fire alarm I described in chapter 2? Well, here it is again—in the form of your body telling you what it *does not want*—but you may not be listening.

Computer technology gave us the metaphor "garbage in, garbage out," as we learned that programming our computers with faulty information would (duh!) result in faulty feedback. In the nutritional world, this same metaphor accurately reflects our dietary habits. For example, too much caffeine or sugar eventually burns you out. On the other hand, protein enhances brain function, and certain types of carbohydrates provide long-term physical endurance.

As a kid, I recall watching Popeye's remarkable diet of spinach, spinach, and more spinach. And boy, did that dude have some muscles on him! My little brother would walk around the house with his spinach stashed in a Tupperware bowl tucked away into his shirt. As he painfully tried to shovel those leafy greens down his throat before attempting some amazing feat of radical strength, he would hyper-salivate, his nostrils would flare, and his eyes would water as he tried not to vomit. But there he was, shoveling that stuff down as best he could, desperate to kick my (or anyone else's) butt any way he could! How that poor child suffered, determined to get those magnificent Popeye muscles. Interestingly enough, though, that 1950s (and earlier) message was right on—spinach *does* make you stronger, and eating it *will* provide critical vitamins and minerals your body needs to thrive. Popeye really did have it going on! These basics have, bit by bit, once again become accepted standard.

What Do the Athletic Superstars Really Eat?

If you really knew what some of our superstar athletes eat, you'd be shocked! For a long time, I watched in amazement as top-ranked tennis and hockey players consumed the most hideous diets. For many, this was simply an uninformed reflection of the cultural diet they were accustomed to from their countries of origin; they simply had *no idea* that this "McDiet" of fries and a shake for breakfast was limiting their athletic competence. Even more astounding was how these amazing athletes could perform so incredibly well despite the destructive smoking and drinking habits they had cultivated over the years.

Fortunately, athletes now pay far closer attention to improving the grade of the fuel they put into their systems. They understand that limiting the quantity of food consumed per sitting is critical, and the dearly departed days of slaughtering a mound of lasagna or chowing down at the buffet station are not only inappropriate but also downright detrimental to great performance. Superstar athletes even know that drinking too much water before a meal can negatively affect their digestion and the way the body trains itself to replace the vital nutrients lost during, say, three grueling hours playing tennis under the blazing sun.

Here's your first tip from "Superstar Athlete Nutrition 101": Our bodies can only digest a certain amount of food at one sitting; eating too much disrupts the body's innate balance and stresses your finely tuned digestive tract, while your body tries to discard the excess that it cannot process. It's like this: if I gave you free gasoline, you would certainly want to top off your tank and save a few bucks, right? But if I offered it to you after your tank was already full, you'd be distraught, as you watched the excess simply spill out onto the ground and go to waste.

DR. BARON'S SUPERSTAR HEALTH TIP:

Our bodies can only digest a certain amount of food at one sitting.

It's the same with your belly; that you are not throwing up isn't, by itself, an indicator that you ate precisely the right amount. If gasoline was spilling onto the floor of the station, you would certainly say, "Oops, too much." But do you know when enough food is enough food? In this era of "supersized" everything, you need to be able to identify how much you should eat at each sitting and when to stop, even if it's your favorite meal. Once you have satisfied your body's requirements for nutrition, the rest just spills over to become fat or an uncomfortable digestive nightmare or the genesis for disease. By the way, did you know that the root of most disease lies in an overloaded colon that has become so packed with gunk it cannot effectively cleanse your body like it is supposed to? Yup—the more you poop, the less you droop! Or, said another way, the more you excrete, the better you compete.

Read on, my friends, and I'll tell you everything you need to know about food, water, and maximum performance.

The Right Fuel for the Right Machine: Eating Right + Drinking Right = Optimal Fitness

Eat, Drink, and be Wary

Proper diet is as critical to an academic using his brain as it is to an athlete using her body. The same nutritional secrets that produce top physical athletic performance also generate top mental performance. Thus, the simple approaches used by professional athletes to enhance their athletic ability will also enhance your ability to score well on a written or verbal test, memorize an equation or a soliloquy, or present a top-notch presentation.

Here's some information about how different substances work in your body and either enhance or prevent your body from achieving its maximum potential.

Liquid Nutritional Secret #1: The Watering Hole

If you drink too much fluid before, during, or after eating, the acids in your stomach that are specifically designed to help you digest your food become less effective and, instead of efficiently breaking down your food to get the most nutritional value, you'll tend to have gas, bloating, cramping, and other delightful symptoms. Sound at all familiar?

It's kind of like this. Have you ever gone camping? You are advised to bring a small amount of bleach to purify your water before drinking it if you are in an area where a questionable water supply may contain harmful bacteria. If you dumped that entire bottle of bleach in your water, you'd probably kill yourself and everyone else who drank the water. Or, at the very least, you'd spend an extremely unpleasant night or two in the nearest hospital having your stomach pumped while you retched uncontrollably. Bleach is not intended to be used full strength for drinking. In this case, you dilute it so it can become *more* effective.

With stomach acids, however, the opposite is true: the more diluted they are, the *less* effective they become. Because the hydrochloric acid in the stomach is responsible for breaking down and assimilating your food, the dilution of these same acids with fluids, juice, cola, coffee, and water will alter the dynamic of the acid and render it ineffective. *Therefore, for the best nutritional assimilation of your food, you should drink your large amounts of fluid 30 minutes prior to eating and 60 minutes postprandial (after a meal).* For maximum effectiveness, you want your stomach acids as intense and concentrated as possible.

Water is essential to our well-being, so I'm by no means suggesting that you shouldn't drink lots and lots of water. On the contrary, I am advocating that you drink *lots*; just pay attention to when, how, and what you are drinking. Our bodies are made up of about 60 percent water, and some organs require as much as 90 percent water to function effectively. Conventional wisdom directing us all to drink "eight 8-ounce glasses of water per day" may not actually be the best advice for properly tending to all our variously sized and shaped bodies. The amount of water we all need varies from person to person. Moreover, how much water we need may also depend on the activity we are performing.

Water is so vital to our survival that men's bathrooms in facilities where athletes can be at high risk for dehydration actually have color charts in every urinal to help identify if an individual is at low, medium, or high risk of dehydration. The way you are asked to do this is by examining the color of your urine (keep your eyes to yourself, boys, it's *your* pee-pee that's the issue here, not your neighbor's!). Actually, this is one of the best methods to see how your body retains or loses fluid so you can be responsible for yourself. Some teams require athletes to weigh in before and after practice to develop their own sixth sense about how much fluid they lose during practice.

Using the chart to assess the color provides a more accurate reflection of hydration status. A color numbered one through three is the target for each player, showing a balanced hydration status. Colors four and five suggest dehydration, and colors six through eight indicate severe dehydration.

[Since the chart is in color, you can access it from the web site: www. drspencerbaron.com. – click on the tab that is titled "Resources" – scroll down to the second page.
You may want to print the chart out to easily identify the color of your urine. Improtant note: 1) Use a color printer 2) You may want to laminate (or cover in plastic) – especially for the guys who tend to miss their target.]

This is true for persons of all ages, abilities, and interests. One United Kingdom school experimented with providing water to students throughout the day and banning carbonated drinks; the school reported improvements in concentration levels, academic performance, and pupil behavior.[16] Teachers in schools taking part in the UK "Food in

---

16   Laura Davis, "Ban on fizzy drinks boosts pupils' work," *icCheshireOn-line.co.uk*, Cheshire: icCheshireOnline, 2003, http://iccheshireonline.icnetwork.

Schools Water Provision Pilot Project" also reported, "The enhanced water provision contributed to a more settled and productive learning environment, as well as helping instill good habits."[17] Moreover, drinking water may reduce tiredness, irritability, and distraction and can have a positive effect on pupils' concentration throughout the day.[18] Finally, the same study reported that children complained less of having headaches and were more aware of the importance of keeping hydrated.[19]

Personally, I used to spend many worried afternoons listening to my son complain of headaches before we identified that there was a direct correlation between his hydration and exertion. Paying close attention to his hydration has allowed me to spend a lot more time enjoying him and his activities and a lot less agony stressing over the impending brain tumor or other horrible disease I imagined he might have. (Before you laugh at me for overreacting like all good and sane parents do, my former sister-in-law did indeed die of a brain tumor, so this is a very real fear for me.)

Liquid Nutritional Secret #2:
Water—It's Not Just for Summer Anymore!

What the heck do I know about fluids and cold weather? After all, I've lived in sunny south Florida since I was eleven years old. We have one of the largest snow ski clubs in the country, and many of my athletes are also skiers. When my athletes trek up north to the frozen tundra, they need to be prepared. Believe it or not, you can dehydrate much more easily in cold weather than in hot.

There are two ways you lose water from your body: perspiration and

---

co.uk/0100news/0100regionalnews/tm_method=full%26objectid=13312972%26si
teid=50020-name_page.html.

17 *Water UK: Working on Behalf of the Water Industry towards a Sustainable Future*, London: Water UK, 2006.

http://www.water.org.uk/home/water-for-health/medical-facts/children.

18 *Food in Schools: Water provision toolkit. Available at:* http://www.healthedtrust.com/indicates/gdhelthinit.htm.

19 J. Almond, *Water in Schools Evaluation.* http://www.water.org.uk/home/water-for-health/news-viewpoint/water-in-schools-in-england-/water-in-schools.pdf

respiration. Here's the thing about perspiration: In hot weather, you know you're sweating and thirsty, and so you drink. Cold weather, on the other hand, impairs your ability to recognize thirst because blood is diverted *away* from the extremities (hands and feet), in toward the core of the body. This is essential to protect the vital organs that are much more important for survival, but it impairs the body's normal approach to identifying and signaling thirst. In cold weather, the actual amount of blood in your body (blood volume) decreases, which causes your hormones to inaccurately convince your organs that they are stable and don't need more water. This can deteriorate far beyond the point where you would normally recognize the warning signals, as in hot weather. And you don't sweat—the most obvious signal that you are losing fluids.

Here's how respiratory fluid loss occurs. When you exhale, you are expelling warm air and fluid from the lungs. In warm weather, the air temperature is comparable to your body's temperature, so you are not aware of the fluid being expelled. In cold weather, however, the cold air causes the droplets of fluid to turn to steam—like when you were a kid and pretending to "smoke" as you exhaled. The same thing occurs in both warm and cold weather, but, in cold weather, you can see it.

This, in itself, does not mean you are losing more fluid; it's just that in cold weather, the fluid loss is more visible. My point is simply that breath is another way the body expels fluid and, in cold weather, you need to replace fluid regularly, even though you don't feel the effects as directly as in summer when you sweat. Moreover, your sweat evaporates more quickly in the cold air, and your body is working harder under the weight of your extra clothing in winter. All of these elements combine to make the threat of dehydration much more acute in cold winter weather than you might expect.

So, don't be lulled into thinking that you don't need to drink as much water in winter as in summer—proper hydration just takes a little more attention and management from you because you don't feel as thirsty. Use the same principles in cold weather as you would in hot: don't wait until you're thirsty; drink fluids continuously; and make sure your urine is clear and not a dark yellow.

Liquid Nutritional Secret #3:
A Nice Cuppa Java Joe

Conventional wisdom used to hold that drinking coffee before any kind of exertion, especially if you were working or playing in the hot, sunny weather, was tantamount to original sin. This logic held that caffeine's diuretic properties would facilitate fluid elimination rather than retention and that, as vital nutrients necessary for normal physical activity were lost, the body might simultaneously overheat like a car without radiator fluid. Dehydration might also even cause a small but critical shrinkage of the tissue around the brain that could result in significant coordination problems.[20] So, over the years, coffee was not only considered a definite no-no, but too much caffeine in the diet before some professional events was banned due to its ergogenic (performance-enhancing) effect.

But, guess what?! *Big news*: COFFEE BEFORE COMPETITION IS NOW CONSIDERED SAFE!

The latest research has found that drinking coffee before a practice or an event could actually *help* with hydration and that moderate coffee consumption only produces very limited risk of dehydration or hyperthermia (overheating).[21] Let me be *very* clear here: I am *not* referring to pills or any other form of artificially processed caffeine; I'm *only* talking about caffeine in the form of a nice, big old cuppa Joe. Cool, huh?

Now, just to put this in perspective, this does not mean you should go out and down as many Starbuck's venti double espresso lattes as possible. Indeed, coffee is still number one on the hit list of what to avoid for anyone trying to balance his or her health, irrespective of athletic performance—it has a pH of 4. This means that it increases

---

20   M-M. G. Wilson and J. E. Morley, "Impaired cognitive function and mental performance in mild dehydration," *European Journal of Clinical Nutrition* 57 (Suppl 2) (2003): S24–S29.
21   L. E. Armstrong, D. J. Casa, C. M. Maresh, and M. S. Ganio, "Caffeine, Fluid-Electrolyte Balance, Temperature Regulation, and Exercise-Heat Tolerance," *Exercise Sport Science Review* 35(3) (2007): 135–40.

the acidity in your body, which makes it more difficult for your body to eliminate toxins, which increases the likelihood of disease and dysfunction.

Other popular drinks also increase your body's acidity. For example, beer has a pH of 2.5; soft drinks carry a pH of 2. In order to neutralize *one* glass of cola, you'd have to drink about *32* glasses of water! The reason you want to decrease how much coffee, soda, beer, and other highly acidic drinks you ingest is that, even though you may not directly observe their harmful effect, they can reduce the body's ability to deal with the digestion and absorption of necessary minerals, specifically calcium, which is critically important for muscular contraction. Don't get confused; I did say earlier that coffee is OK, but remember that the key to using any potentially harmful substance is always *moderation.*

Liquid Nutritional Secret #4:
The Gatorade Crusade

Gatorade and other electrolyte-replacement drinks are terrific for helping you replace essential nutrients lost during rigorous exercise. But here's the thing about Gatorade: it isn't a nice soft drink or juice substitute for folks who sit around, so don't use it that way! When Gatorade started appearing in public school and other vending machines right next to the soda pop, it became popular as a tasty, noncarbonated soda alternative. Great for company profits; not so great for your body. Gatorade was, and still is, meant for the active body to help it replenish fluids and vital nutrients that are lost through perspiration, urination, and intensified body function during exercise. Gatorade was never intended for inactive, sedentary individuals, as the extra calories consumed but not used after this or any bottle of "electrolyte-replacement" drink, will be completely wasted. They'll just make you fat. The *only* time to use Gatorade or something similar if you are not vigorously exercising is after a bad case of Montezuma's Revenge (for those who have never been to Mexico, that's a fancy way of saying "diarrhea"), when your body has lost large amounts of fluids and nutrients through the back door, so to speak.

Now that Gatorade and other high-performance endurance drinks are so popular, how do you know which one is best for what you need? Like I said, none of these drinks are meant for the "armchair athlete" or "video football" champs. They are expressly meant to replenish the lost nutrients and electrolytes lost through excessive sweating and should be used to avoid muscle cramping and spasm caused by dehydration. Here are three criteria to help you determine the right drink for you:

1) *Fructose (high-fructose corn syrup) and glucose (sucrose syrup) should be the initial ingredients on the label and should be in a 55 to 45 percent ratio.*
2) *The drink should contain less than 6 percent to 8 percent carbohydrates.*
3) *Sodium content should be approximately 110 grams per 8 ounces.*

Amanda Carlson,
Director of Performance Nutrition and Athlete's Performance,
Consultant to professional and elite athletes

How much you sweat is the indicator for what kind of hydration you need. So, when you are exercising rigorously, lick your arm! Yeah—go ahead—lick your arm! This is how you can tell if you are a "salty sweater," which will determine what kind of drink you need. If you have a lot of salt in your sweat, then increase the sodium to 170 to 200 grams per 8 ounces.

Here's a *really* top secret athletic superstar tip: I am under strict oath not to reveal my source here, as it could cause a major upset between the team and its sponsor, who pours tons of money into advertising claims that its company hydrates this team. This secret was accidentally spilled while I was in the locker room of a National Basketball Association team. Get this—even though the team advertises the name of the company on the side of its huge, orange and green drink dispenser, *there is only WATER inside that dispenser*! But it's not just *any* water; it's designed to meet two critical specific hydration criteria for these athletes:

1. *It must be room temperature* so the body does not have to work as hard warming it down to the body's temperature. Warming the water takes vital energy from the body.
2. *The water must be high-alkaline (that is, have a high pH balance).* As such, the preferred brand is Fiji (as per this strength coach).

Summary

Here's a recap of my Liquid Nutritional Secrets. The most important thing to remember is that you *must* hydrate your body and you must use the right hydration for the right activity. Water is always essential and, when exercising rigorously, be sure to remember to replace the vitamins and nutrients you have lost thorough your sweat.

> ***Liquid Nutritional Secret #1: The Watering Hole.*** Drink lots, just not 30 minutes before or sixty minutes after your meal.

> ***Liquid Nutritional Secret #2: Water—It's Not Just for Summer Anymore!*** Be sure to drink plenty in cold weather, when the risk of unintentional dehydration escalates.

> ***Liquid Nutritional Secret #3: A Nice Cuppa Java Joe.*** A good old cup of coffee may enhance your performance.

> ***Liquid Nutritional Secret #4: The Gatorade Crusade.*** Gatorade is great, but use only as directed—not as a juice or soft drink substitute.

Remember, for a beautiful ready-to-print list, check the website and click on "Secret list" for your own copy.

Because we know that men (and women) cannot live on water alone, in chapter 7, I'll give you some top dietary nutritional secrets that will help you identify and maintain the right nutrition for your peak performance body.

Chapter 7

THE ESSENTIAL ATHLETE:

Ultimate Food and
Nutritional Supplement Strategies

*Over the past year, I have closely examined the way my
body reacts to many different foods. Most importantly, in
the way of blood sugar, energy, and hunger. It's crucial to
find what works best for your body. Protein keeps me full
and mentally sharp. I often drink green tea, eat organic
protein bars or a protein shake during a round. I do not
try new foods before a tournament round.*
Natalie Gulbis, LPGA Golfer

The next important thing for us to discuss is how to manage your
diet for optimal results. Superstar athletes manage their food and
nutritional supplements rigorously; they cannot perform to the degree
necessary to sustain those multimillion-dollar contracts if they do not
take proper care of their bodies. A performance-enhancing diet is one of

the simplest and most important elements an athlete must integrate to stay in top shape and get those contracts signed by the highest bidder.

As I already spent enough time telling you basic rules about how to understand diet and nutrition in chapter 6, I won't waste space here, and I'll just get right to the meat of the matter—how to eat right to keep your body tight.

Eating Right

Eating right is one of the most important and most basic concepts necessary to enhance peak performance. It's so obvious, most of us don't think about it all that much; we just do what feels right. In fact, nutrition is so vital to the professional athlete that, whenever major league baseball's Philadelphia Phillies, New York Yankees, and Milwaukee Brewers travel to play at the home of an opposing team, the host team's clubhouse manager is formally requested to please:

➢ Remove all sweets.
➢ Do not serve fried foods.
➢ Use 100 percent beef hot dogs only.
➢ Provide only diet soda.
➢ Offer pizza with cheese only—no toppings.
➢ Serve only baked chips.

These very basic rules make a major impact on how well the million-dollar bodies of these superstar athletes perform. Only makes sense that you should abide by these same rules, doesn't it?

Here are some ways to consciously manage what goes into your body before it goes into athletic overdrive.

Food and Nutritional Supplement Secret #1: Switch-Hit Your Foods for Peak Performance

---

Have you ever experienced a runny nose, excess mucous in your throat, watery eyes, scratchy throat, headache, or itchy skin after you eat—sometimes after only the first few bites? Researchers are noting a growing phenomenon called "food sensitivity," which is different from the more obvious full-blown allergic reaction you might easily recognize. Rather, it is a much more subtle reaction to some substance (natural or synthetic) in your food. It often happens with foods you eat frequently.

As creatures of habit, we often eat the same things *a lot*. As we do this, our bodies tend to lose the ability to break down and digest those same foods over time. The inability to properly digest food can also result from inflammation of the lining around the digestive system, or gut, which may be due to excess caffeine, alcohol, stress, or chemicals in food, such as aspartame. Another symptom of poor digestion is bad breath; your body gradually becomes incapable of effectively dissolving and assimilating that same food efficiently over and over again (of course, your skanky breath may simply be from all that garlic and onion you just ate or the six Cosmopolitans you drank last night).

The cheapest, easiest, and most effective way to test what's going on with you and your food is to journal your reactions to certain foods; then you can simply eliminate the bad ones from your diet. Believe it or not, sometimes, eliminating these ritualistically eaten foods from your diet may even cause symptoms similar to drug withdrawal! But the upside is that you will feel healthier and more energetic, as your body no longer struggles to process foods it cannot effectively manage.

A costlier but more accurate approach is a "food sensitivity test," which requires drawing blood. The blood is then sent to a lab and tested against some 200 different foods to identify an immune system reaction. An easy-to-read color chart—where you can see that foods falling into the red category are prohibited, foods in the amber category are cautioned, and foods in the green category should be eaten regularly every third day, shows the results. Be cautioned, however, as several of my NFL football player patients took themselves off the diet because *one of the side effects was weight loss*! While this was a problem for these guys, who need all that extra bulk, for most of us, that would be just fine, wouldn't it?!

> # *Food and Nutritional Supplement Secret #2: Chow Down!*

How many times did your mother warn you not to go swimming for an hour after you ate because you'd get "cramps"? Meanwhile, you sullenly watched all your friends play while you just sat there— miserable, embarrassed, and *hot*. So what is this "cramp" thing anyway? Why does it happen? And was Mom actually right?

The reason that you would cramp while swimming right after eating is that the muscles used for playing compete for blood flow with the muscles needed for digestion. Neither set of muscles functions effectively without a sufficient blood supply pumped in to help them work. Not surprisingly, the strong muscles used for sports will always win this competition and shunt the blood away from your digestive tract, making it harder for you to process your food. Thus, if you exercise right after eating, the food does not digest effectively, and you cramp. Your mom rightly feared that if you swam too soon after eating, you just might drown because you cramped in the deep water. Sorry, but Mom *was* on target. Now, as an adult, if you cramp on the court or field, you can just bend over and puke it all up. Not pretty, but at least you won't die.

Just as I was writing this, I took a break to go get my eight-year-old son ready for his soccer game. I saw him finishing a bowl of pasta in butter sauce, followed by a glazed doughnut. Like the good, not-too-overbearing dad I aspire to be, I kept my mouth firmly shut, despite my concern. Moreover, I did not want to be responsible for predisposing him to anticipate, and thus create, his own discomfort that might jeopardize his performance. I decided to hold my tongue until the end of the game; it was important he know about how to eat properly, but, like all great moments, timing is everything. As expected, at midgame, I saw him grab the area underneath his lower right ribs and hold it while he dribbled the ball. At the quarter, he glumly acknowledged he was cramping—further confirmation that Mama's intuition about poor pregame nutrition was correct.

To overcome the problem of needing to eat before you exercise, there are now many nutritionally engineered food bars (like Power Bars, not martini bars!) and drinkable, nutritious shakes that allow you to get good energy close to your event or practice time without the heaviness or digestive challenges of a full meal. These are great, nutritious substitutes for a bowl of pasta and an ice cream chaser. I eat them all the time. This same principle applies to cognitive sports like auto racing or low physical activity sports like chess. The idea is to have the most blood flowing to your brain and the least amount in the digestive system. Here's my evidence for this theory; I dare you to compete in a spelling bee after a Thanksgiving dinner!

I will never forget being in the Miami Dolphins training room and consistently observing a finely tuned, muscular professional athlete take the team's handheld, industrial-strength massage vibrator and bury it into his abdomen after each meal. Inquiring mind that I have, I had ask *what the heck he was doing.* As he was my patient, I was concerned that he had neglected to tell me about some injury that was bothering him. To my surprise, he said, "Nope, Doc, nothing's wrong, just easin' my digestion." By his logic, this postprandial regime enhanced his ability to digest his food prior to football practice.

Did this make sense to me? Well, once I thought about it, I reasoned that perhaps this low-level vibration increased the blood flow to the area where he most needed it—his digestive tract—which in turn helped his body better assimilate his food. Remember how exercise following a meal circulates blood away from the digestive organs into the muscles, thus impairing digestion and increasing stomach cramps? Well, this gentle "belly massage" does just the opposite. Try it and see if it works for you.

Not all athletes have the same strategies. The trick is to find out what works best for your body and then develop an ongoing strategy so your body can derive the most strength and energy for your particular sport. Here's what a couple of the most nutritionally fit athletes eat before an event:

> On my day to start ... it's better for me to eat pasta or sometimes rice and beans. I never eat [a] meat before the start. In Cuba, it was only rice and beans. Our nutritionist said this was the best!
>
> **Orlando "El Duque" Hernandez**, pitcher, New York Mets

Fish is good brain food. Therefore, before or during the tournament week, I eat salmon or swordfish with steamed vegetables.

Natalie Gulbis, LPGA Golfer

Supplements and Household Remedies

In addition to how you eat, what else you put in your precious body is also extremely important to both your overall well-being and as your athletic performance. Some of the most important secrets to peak performance lie in nutritional supplements and household remedies that are fast, easy, cheap, and very accessible. Here are a few tips on how to make the most of what you can find at your local health food store, drugstore, or even what's already in your kitchen pantry or bathroom medicine chest.

Food and Nutritional Supplement Secret #3: Stop Dragging, Start GAG-ging!

Does your body sometimes just hurt for no apparent reason? Do your muscles or joints ache, and you can't seem to figure out the cause? Well, there is a supplement that can ease your discomfort without much effort on your part. It's a vitamin supplement called glucosamine chondroitin that athletes, certified athletic trainers, and health-care professionals are increasingly using to help minimize pain and inflammation, expand range of motion in osteoarthritis patients, and repair damaged cartilage. Glucosamine chondroitin works by increasing the production of glycosaminoglycans (GAGs for short), and here's why glucosamine and chondroitin are important and how they work.

Cartilage is a valuable lining that covers joint surfaces, much like Teflon does a cooking pan. The preservation of cartilage is vitally important to the professional (or any) athlete's safety and physical longevity; this is why many locker rooms have these supplements (also called glucosamine hydrochloride and chondroitin sulfate) readily available for their athletes to consume, especially as a preventive measure.

Cartilage cells (chondrocytes) produce important components of cartilage called glycosaminoglycans (GAGs) and proteoglycans (PGs). PGs (and the GAGs they are made of) can hold large amounts of water, which allows cartilage to provide cushioning, resist compression, and absorb shock. In order to make GAGs and PGs, chondrocytes must first make glucosamine and chondroitin. By ingesting supplemental forms of these accessory nutrients, cartilage production is more efficient (which is especially important in the aging body) because it takes fewer steps to repair and/ or rebuild GAGs and PGs. An analogy is the difference between making hotcakes from a water-only mix versus one requiring milk, eggs, and oil. If you take glucosamine, just add water and you'll be cooking.

Dr. Doug Andersen,
Diplomat American
Chiropractic Board of Sports Physicians;
Certified Clinical Nutritionist;
Former medical director for the
Association of Volleyball Professionals;
Former nutrition consultant to the Los Angeles Kings

A 2006 study funded by the National Center for Complementary and Alternative Medicine (NCCAM) and the National Institute of Arthritis and Musculoskeletal and Skin Diseases examined the effects of this supplement on osteoarthritic patients. The study concluded that "[T]he combination of glucosamine and chondroitin sulfate may be effective in the subgroup of patients with moderate to severe knee pain."[22] While this may not sound like a resounding endorsement, what is most important to note here is that the *government* funded and

---

22   D. O. Clegg, D. J. Reda, C. L. Harris, M. A. Klein, J. R. O'Dell, M. M. Hooper, J. D. Bradley, et al., "Glucosamine, chondroitin sulfate, and the two in combination for painful knee osteoarthritis," *New England Journal of Medicine* 354 (2006): 795–808.

conducted this study. In other words, the government is now tacitly acknowledging the impact and effectiveness of this supplement; it no longer resides solely in the realm of "alternative" medicine used primarily by nonmainstream health-care practitioners. That, my friends, is good news indeed.

Food and Nutritional Supplement Secret #4: Arm & Hammer your Sore Muscles!

I wonder if the Arm & Hammer baking soda folks know that their refrigerator freshener, cleaning, and cooking product can also be used for sore muscles? If you are not inclined to popping pills when discomfort arises, a touch of good old-fashioned baking soda may be a cheap and easy way to reduce the fatigue, burn, and pain of a sore muscle during anaerobic activity (this is different and not to be confused with the muscle soreness you feel 24 to 48 hours after exercise). A very small recent study showed that ingesting sodium bicarbonate before exercise effectively buffered the pH balance of the blood before and during a sprint test.[23] In essence, this means that the lactic acid your body produced during rigorous exercise, which created that "burning feeling" is reduced by taking baking soda before exercising. Now, don't go all hog wild here and start downing boxes of baking soda; more is definitely not better, and too much will give you stomach cramps and diarrhea. However, in small doses, it may be useful, especially if you haven't exercised in a while or are trying a new activity. Some "gym rats" recommend a tablespoon of baking soda in a glass of water before altering and increasing the intensity of your usual routine (or no more than 1 tablespoon per 180 pounds of bodyweight). A similar effect might be realized by taking an Alka-Seltzer prior to a indulging in a new, more rigorous routine.

---

23   David Bishop and Brett Claudius, "Effects of Induced Metabolic Alkalosis on Prolonged Intermittent-Sprint Performance," *Medicine and Science in Sports and Exercise* 37, 5 (2005): 759–67.

Food and Nutritional Supplement Secret #5: Chicken Soup (and More) for the Body ... or, Sometimes Mama Really Does Know Best!

Ever wonder what made that big, bruising, 240-pound, bone-crushing defensive lineman into the beast that he is today? Often, he credits his mama's home remedies as the source of his greatness. These anecdotal stories are fun and sometimes surprisingly more significant than you might think. And why do you think these multimillion-dollar athletes, whose incomes depend on staying well, follow these remedies?

Because Mama said so, of course!

Growing up in a Jewish family, in my home, all ills were cured by a hearty bowl (or two or three!) of Mom's homemade chicken soup. When nothing else tasted good or made me feel better, this stuff really worked! While some might attribute the curative qualities of chicken soup to lots of love and folklore, recent evidence has indeed verified its medicinal effect. Research has shown that this remarkable concoction of chicken, onions, sweet potatoes, parsnips, turnips, carrots, celery, parsley, salt, and pepper (at least that's how my mom made it) actually enhances your blood cells' ability to fight infection, as well as produce an amino acid called cysteine, which boosts the respiratory system; the steam eases the mucous buildup in the nose.[24] Amazing, huh?

One athlete used to tell me how his auntie would wrap freshly cut tobacco leaves around his badly bruised and banged up body. The bruises would go away almost instantly. I mostly just found this mildly amusing, until I read about how tobacco is considered one of the most important plants used by tribes in the northwest Amazon. Tobacco is used in curative rituals by rubbing a concentrated substance from the leaves briskly over sprains and bruises. Fresh leaves can also be crushed

---

24
B. O. Rennard, R. F. Ertl, and G. L. Gossman, R. A. Robbins, and S. I. Rennard, "Chicken soup inhibits neutrophil chemotaxis *in vitro*," *Chest* 118 (2000) 1150–57.

and made into a soft, moist mass known as a poultice and placed over boils and infected wounds.[25] Who knew?!

In my years spent behind locker room doors, I've spotted some pretty interesting poultices used in the back rooms of some of the most prestigious training facilities. You won't see these on any TV commercial; they are gifts from Mother Earth. Not worth large pharmaceutical company backing, they could put quite a dent in big pharma profits if used regularly. Nutritionists, homeopaths, acupuncturists, chiropractors, and even some medical doctors have personal witches' brews that bring out the best in human performance.

I know some athletes who regularly request the services of a Doctor of Oriental Medicine who, in addition to traditional acupuncture practices, also utilizes a completely different methodology of examination, diagnosis, and treatment than we are accustomed to receiving by our Western-trained medical doctors. As per Asian medical dictates, many conditions can be treated by cooking up a fantastic brew of roots, branches, herbs, and other shrubbery to be sipped as a (rather nasty-tasting) tea.

Such herbal concoctions are designed to heal the organs and glands—in the case of the concoction below, the adrenals, small glands that sit atop each kidney and manufacture the hormones that control how you metabolize fats, proteins, and carbohydrates. Your adrenals also assist your immune system, aid in reducing inflammation, and help you cope with physical and emotional stress. An herbal brew designed to strengthen this important, yet often neglected, body part contains Siberian ginseng, borage, huang qi, and the eye of newt (OK, just kidding about the last one).

The key in Chinese medicine is to care for the organs *before* conditions manifest into bigger and more unruly diseases. A common misconception about Chinese medicine is that it is a "strategy of last resort" when someone is already in the worst way and has exhausted all the more traditional options. This is often how allopathic medicine is administered. Rather, Chinese methods focus on identifying conditions long before they can be seen on the Western "radar screen" of blood lab evaluations and other expensive tests. Instead, Chinese doctors look at

---

25   R. E. Schultes and R. F. Raffauf, *The Healing Forest: Medicinal and Toxic Plants of the Northwest Amazonia*, (Portland: Dioscorides Press, 1995).

the texture and color of your skin, its surrounding tissue, your eyes, your tongue, and six different pulses on your wrists that correspond with different regions of the body. They are very sensitive to the body's warning signs, and hence, able to identify and suppress disease long before it becomes unmanageable, and generally long before a standard Western-trained doctor might notice it.

Here's an example of someone I know who tried this route, though, in typical Western fashion, long after her condition had already become critical. I have a good friend whose badly ruptured disc threatened to paralyze her from the waist down, as it was compressing the nerves in her lower spine (for all you medical buffs out there, it's called Cauda Equina Syndrome). After several months of debilitating pain and many doctors' visits, she awoke one morning to find she could barely stand up and was rapidly losing all sensation from the waist down. She was also losing bladder function and was unable to urinate, despite her painful and urgent need to go. Her doctor ordered an ambulance rushed to her home, and she was admitted to the hospital for emergency microsurgery that morning. Following the surgery, she was fortunate to recover full use of her legs but was left with a paralyzed bladder, requiring permanent catheterization and significant remaining numbness from her groin down through the back of her thighs. While in the hospital, she was taught how to self-catheterize and was put on permanent daily antibiotics to minimize the risk of infection. She was 34 at the time.

Determined not to spend the rest of her life urinating through a tube, she embarked on a rigorous journey through a variety of alternative treatments. She developed a routine that included acupuncture several times a week and nightly cooking of oriental herbs prescribed by a rather scary Asian man in a dark back room. The herbs tasted so bad she had to put gobs of honey in the brew just to get it down. She carried this brew everywhere and drank it for months. (Ever see the episode of *Sex and the City* where Charlotte goes to New York City's Chinatown into a mysterious, dark back room to see an Oriental doctor for herbs to help her get pregnant? It was *just* like that.)

After ten months of following her treatment routine (though she had dropped the acupuncture a few months before), her bladder began to function again. When she called her doctor to say her bladder function was returning, he was happy for her but skeptical. He monitored her closely for some time, as she got better and better. It is now some years later, and she remains fully recovered (though still has some remaining numbness).

You know what her doctor finally said before he discharged her completely? He had never told her, but he had been pretty certain she would *never* recover—not in ten months and not in ten years. While he had not wanted to dampen her enthusiasm, he was quite sure that she would never fully recover and that she would eventually just have to come to terms with the fact that using a self-administered catheter was not the worst thing in the world. At least she could walk and function.

To this day, she remains 100 percent convinced that those herbs and needles altered the course of her life. What's even more amazing is that this is not an isolated case; I have seen several extraordinary stories like this over the years. I share this one because my friend was not a superstar athlete, nor a well-trained health professional, nor anyone with resources that made her any different from any of you reading this book. She was an average, 34-year-old woman living in New York City. The only difference between you and her may be her tenacity and persistence. These qualities, however, were brought on by what she perceived to be the gravity of her situation; she was bound and determined not to be stopped by what some doctor told her (or didn't tell her, in this case). You are exactly the same and have exactly the same resources, intelligence, and capacity.

A Note

For better or worse, stricter standards intended to eliminate the use of "performance-enhancing" substances have caused athletes to be considerably more cautious about what they ingest. Not only are the penalties becoming increasingly severe, but also many "natural" products have been found to have traces of "controlled substances" that, if detected, could have disastrous legal and financial consequences for athletes. For the pro athlete, just one positive test begins the unpleasant and time-consuming task of urinating in a cup on a regular basis. Some athletes have to be tested as often as *three times a week*.

Interestingly, there is still no reliable test for human growth hormone on the market, despite its use as one of the more effective performance-enhancing drugs in existence. Moreover, there are some nutritional supplements that include comparable substances to stimulate growth hormones that would not be on the list of banned substances because they are not monitored by WADA, the World Anti-Doping Agency, which governs many major sports, including the Olympic Games. (For a list of banned substances visit: http://www.wada-ama.org/en/prohibitedlist.ch2). Drug monitoring is an emerging area that continues to shift almost as quickly as you can say "controlled substance." Much of the information on the Internet is not up-to-date or reliable, so be careful what you read on the World Wide Web. For a regularly updated list of what's "in" and what's "out," be sure to check my website at www.DrSpencerBaron.com for the most current information.

Summary

We've now covered the secrets used by many professional athletes to enhance their performance, using basic nutritional guidance. As always, you'll find these in a beautiful and easy-to-download form on my website, www.DrSpencerBaron.com. I'll be updating the list regularly, so check back often. Here's what we've covered in chapter 7:

Food and Nutritional Supplement Secret #1: Switch-Hit Your Foods for Peak Performance. Regularly alternate your food so your body doesn't become overly accustomed to the same diet.

Food and Nutritional Supplement Secret #2: Chow Down! Don't eat too much at a single meal; respect your body's limits.

Food and Nutritional Supplement Secret #3: Stop Dragging, Start GAG-ging. Use glucosamine chondroitin, the precursor to the glycosaminoglycans (GAGs) to help decrease pain and inflammation, increase range of motion, and repair damaged cartilage.

Food and Nutritional Supplement Secret #4: Arm & Hammer Your Sore Muscles. Take a small amount of baking soda before your workout to help minimize muscle soreness.

Food and Nutritional Supplement Secret #5: Chicken Soup (and More) for the Body ... or, Sometimes Mama Really Does Know Best. Seek out and use great home remedies; they really work.

Now that we've covered mental and nutritional secrets of the superstar athletes, let's move on to the last side of the triangle that I showed you in chapter 1. In chapter 8, I'll show you powerful physical secrets that will complete your treasure chest of secrets to peak performance and powerful well-being.

(Just as with the mental secrets, enter the code ENERGY on my website, www.DrSpencerBaron.com, and I'll give you three more great nutritional secrets to help accelerate your progress!)

Chapter 8:

THE ESSENTIAL ATHLETE:

Ultimate Physical Strategies for *Overall* Body Healing, Strength, and Conditioning

So far, you've read about some of the best mental and nutritional secrets of the superstar athletes. Sports fan or not, finding out what superstar athletes, who have the best health care in the world, do to stay in peak condition is invaluable. My hope and intention are that this information inspires you to take a new level of responsibility for your own health and well-being, irrespective of what your insurance allows, your overworked and burned-out doctor offers (or fails to offer), or whatever "late, breaking news" there is about some recent study that proves (or disproves) the benefits (or dangers) of whatever drugs your body has become dependent on. I am well aware of how confusing the market out there is; the best thing you can do is become your own greatest advocate and resource. That's what I see as my job— empowering you to be your own best caretaker by knowing when to help yourself and when to get help from others.

The next step in our journey together is to understand the general physical secrets that enable professional athletes to stay healthy, maintain peak performance, and achieve their intended results. While you see amazingly powerful displays of physical grace and ability on television or at live events, you rarely hear about what goes on behind the scenes to ensure that image. The intense physical training and rehabilitation that the athlete undergoes to surpass his or her own limits while simultaneously entertaining you may defy whatever you used to think about health and healing. Their feats may seem superhuman, but they are really just a remarkable combination of creativity, innovation, and knowing how to manage the body to support an environment for excellent health.

Some of this information is so basic and simple that it's distressing that some health-care professionals don't know about it. As a result, it has become my passion to bring all these various health-care disciplines together to offer you the best and most comprehensive array of approaches, in a manner that is easy to understand and simple to follow.

Despite my passion for health care and athletics, I must admit that, after twenty-three years in practice, I have become somewhat impervious to many of the remarkable treatments that grace my daily experience. It's like knowing a language so well that you forget you are speaking it and that others don't understand the words. There is a tendency for me to forget how valuable this information can be, until I become very present to the impact of how these amazing athletes inspire, motivate, and captivate their fans and what it takes to keep them healthy. It is not until I bring a friend or another doctor with me into the locker room treatment site that I realize how blessed I am to be part of this world of innovative and cutting-edge health-care practice. Read on as I share with you some of the wonders of modern health-care practice that rarely get past the locker room door.

General Physical Secret #1:
Going Hot and Cold ... Not Fickle, Just Sensible!

Are you confused about when to use heat and when to use cold after an injury? Welcome to my world; heat versus cold application is one of the simplest care strategies, and at the same time, it's one of the most confusing, and people get hung up by it. Quite frankly, this information isn't even hidden behind the locker room doors; it's right out there in the open. Just take a quick gander at any sporting event to see the bags of ice that are piled onto any injury the minute it happens.

So what's most effective in the first minutes of almost any injury? *Ice it, baby!* In the first moments after an injury, always ice it down.

When do you use heat? When the first 72 hours have passed following a traumatic injury, such as a strain or sprain, you are free to use heat. In most cases of a strain and/or sprain, the athlete uses ice for ten minutes then removes the pack and rests at room temperature for ten minutes then reapplies ice for another ten minutes. This protocol is repeated every two hours. Use this intervention for the first 72 hours following injury.[26] Think of it this way: *Spring always follows winter, and the heat always follows the chill.* This treatment will decrease muscle spasms and pain, while increasing vasoconstriction (shrinking of the swelling blood vessels). Moreover, cold also reduces your sensitivity to pain and the destruction of surrounding tissues.

As elemental as this advice is, I am often surprised how many people don't know what to do. What's even more overwhelming is how many people have ended up in my office after a visit to the hospital emergency room where someone told them to go home and put a hot pack on the injury. This single action just doubled their downtime and kept them injured longer!

What you don't see behind the locker room doors is how the athlete prepares for an event and cares for the part of his or her body that is most active (and likely to be injured) during his or her game; for example, a baseball pitcher would concentrate on his pitching arm and, specifically, his shoulder. "Warming up" entails some crucial preparation that quite literally warms the soon-to-be stressed area. One time, a friend accompanied me during a treatment session for the San Francisco Giants baseball team. My friend was spellbound to see the 6'5" frame of Jason Schmidt with his right shoulder and elbow wrapped in large, hot, moist packs. Through the mist, Schmidt seemed

26   C. M. Bleakley, S. M. McDonough, and D. C. MacAuley, "Cryotherapy for acute ankle sprains: A randomized controlled study of two different icing protocols," *British Journal of Sports Medicine* 40 (2006): 700–705.

to be wrapped in majestic armor, as if he were a white knight preparing to joust. My fascinated friend asked, "Wow, what's that all about?"

I replied, "Oh, he's just 'warming up' his shoulder."

By sending heat to the area, a significant amount of blood flow is directed to a focal area to bathe the muscles, tendons, and ligaments in all the nutrients needed to protect the joint as best as possible. This is done just before the player engages in a low-intensity action such as pregame warm-up in the bullpen prior to full-on pitching.

General Physical Secret #2:
Don't Just Ice It—RICE It!

No, this is not about a heaping helping of Uncle Ben's before you work out (Ugh, my stomach hurts just thinking about that). "RICE" is an acronym for Rest, Ice, Compression, and Elevation, and it's how to care for an injured area to reduce swelling in the first 72 hours following an injury. In addition to a mere bag of ice, which can be awkward and clumsy to manage and get in just the right spot, here's what the professionals actually do:

1) Fill a paper or Styrofoam cup with water and put it in the freezer.

2) When the cup has hardened, peel half an inch of Styrofoam off the rim you have a layer of ice exposed.

3) Using the Styrofoam-covered part of the cup as your handle (you can wrap it in a paper towel for added comfort if you like), place a regular towel under the body part you are going to ice down (for the purpose of soaking up melted ice) and slowly move the cup over the injured area in a continuous motion. This is called "ice massage" and is the preferred way to cool down an injury because it maximizes patient comfort while also

gradually cooling the area, rather than dumping ice all on one spot, which can be extremely uncomfortable.

4) Using the remaining ice cup, fill with preferred brand for a quick Scotch on the rocks.

5) Just kidding.

General Physical Secret #3:
S-T-R-E-T-C-H It Out.

Can you lengthen shortened muscles? When a muscle shortens, it becomes tight, which increases the potential for injury when it then gets lengthened (or stretched) with activity. This is why hamstring muscles (found at the back of your leg, connecting from the buttock to behind the knee) tend to be so prone to injury. Because we spend so much time sitting (most of us do), the hamstring muscle contracts into a shortened state. Over time, the muscle itself starts to accommodate for that position and has a more difficult time lengthening to accommodate activity. When you stand, walk, or run, the muscle stretches. Over time, muscles that are not stretched actually shrink, particularly following injury (this is especially true following a fracture when the body part is casted and must remain immobile for a long period).

Want more muscle length and flexibility? The ideal approach to lengthening contracted muscles is through applying *moist* heat. Dry heat (like that of a heating pad or electric blanket) is less effective. After 15 to 20 minutes of moist heat, stretch the muscle. Then, after a few stretches, take your thumbs and massage them into the muscle. After a couple of minutes, heat the area again for 15 minutes. Repeat the process with massage and some deeper pressure along the whole belly of the muscle. Now, in that stretched position, put an ice pack or use your ice cup and cool the area down. Keep it that way for 15 minutes. If you repeat the cycle a couple times a week, you will begin to add more flexibility and length to the muscle, thus making it less prone to injury.

I'll tell you, with a relatively small 5'5" frame, I sure do wish I could s-t-r-e-t-c-h my muscles to reach my dad's and brother's vantage points of over 6 feet. Unfortunately, that's not the way this works.

The most dramatic example of how muscles shorten is what happens when a woman consistently wears high heels. When she later wears flat shoes or goes barefoot, it is not uncommon for her to overstretch her calf muscle, which then tears like paper. You can spot a candidate for this type of injury when you see her walk without shoes and still look like a ballerina "on point." If you walk on your toes and are uncomfortable with your heels touching the floor, you are a perfect candidate for muscle lengthening as described above.

General Physical Secret #4:
Rubber—It's Not Just for Tires Anymore

If you have never used a piece of rubber (or surgical) tubing while exercising, you are truly missing out on one of life's small pleasures. The versatility of rubber tubing makes it a nice addition to any muscle-strengthening program. It is also especially valuable for those of you who have had the misfortune of getting terminated from your rehabilitation program following surgery or an injury because your health insurance deemed you either "well" or undeserving of further reimbursement.

The other nice thing about rubber tubing is that it eliminates all your excuses about not being able to exercise when you're traveling. You can easily throw this exercise equipment in your luggage and not tip the scales at baggage check-in.

Better yet, "armchair athletes" can use rubber tubing while watching a sporting event on TV and give new meaning to the term *spectator sport*! For your biceps, stand on the tube while curling your arms up and down (it's better than curling beer cans). You can also try grabbing the tube closer to your feet with your arms straight and then squat up and down to strengthen your legs. For your back, try holding onto the tubing with your hands about shoulder-width apart, and then push your hands away from each other, to strengthen your back while also improving your posture. There are many, many exercises you can do with rubber tubing for just about every body part. You can adjust the resistance simply by holding the tube looser or more tautly. A great online resource for a variety of exercises using rubber tubing is Thera-Brand, located at http://www.thera-band.com.

General Physical Secret #5:
Conversion to Inversion

The spine and hips are among the most important weight-bearing joints in the body. These joints take a beating just fighting the gravitational forces, which are always pulling them down, down, down, that they contend with on a daily basis. While this is good stress and ultimately makes them strong, it can also overwhelm these joints so that they deteriorate faster than normal. After some intense pounding from basketball, football, tennis, or gymnastics, for example, you may find your body begging for some relief.

One of the best preventive measures you can take is to hang upside down like a bat on a daily basis. Do you remember how the actor Richard Gere hung upside down with his inversion boots in the 1980 movie *American Gigolo*? While he started a national fad, problems with blood pressure, glaucoma, too much strain on the ankles, and the sudden shock to the spinal cord joints when standing back into the upright position, required significant adjustments be made to the process to ensure it would be safe for everyday use. These subsequent modifications resulted in the *inversion table* for home use. A table allows considerably more control of how fast, how long, to what degree, and how easy it is to hang yourself (upside down, that is). You can find a variety of tables, at varying prices and qualities, by searching online.

Here's my inversion table story. One of my most remarkable experiences was with one of those crazy, extreme athletes who made an ironman triathlon look like a walk in the park. This guy would not only compete for *hours* at a time but for *days* at a time. He was an intelligent man who worked as a pilot and who, rarely if ever, complained of discomfort.

One day, he came in looking like a human question mark and

complaining (mildly) of major low back pain. This day, he simply said, "OK, Doc, fix me up! Whaddya think—a day or two?"

I said I'd do my best and proceeded to examine him. After the exam, his discomfort appeared to be much worse than the usual strains and sprains he typically brought with him, and I felt we should try a two-week, intense treatment and then reevaluate.

"Steve," I asked, "so how did you do this? Flying off your bike or falling from a cliff?"

"No," Steve responded. "I was painting the baseboards around my house and, when I was done, I couldn't straighten up."

Knowing himself as such a superb athlete, Steve was embarrassed about this severe injury resulting from such a nontraumatic, "sissy" activity. He was so mortified, he even asked me to keep it to myself. (I did … until I wrote this book.)

After I'd conservatively treated Steve for about two weeks, he would seem to get better, but then he'd get worse again. I had a hard time reading Steve, as he never let me know how much pain he was truly in, no matter how many ways I tried to get him to open up to me. We decided to run an MRI.

We were both absolutely shocked at the results. Steve had injured not just one, not just two, not even three of his lower spinal cord discs. Indeed, *all five discs* of his low back were pretty severely impaired; three discs were herniated, and two were bulging. That's like coming out of the supermarket and finding four flat tires on your car. Steve's superhuman athletic ego was pretty near crushed. After he resigned himself to the fact that he would not only be unable to race for an entire season, he would also have to ask his airline for, at minimum, a one-month sick leave. In addition, we had to considerably re-strategize our approach to getting him well.

Chiropractic care alone would clearly be insufficient at this point. Steve would have to do something every day, a few times a day. I suggested an inversion table as an adjunct to what we were doing in the office. Since surgery would have been his other alternative, he was committed to trying anything before entertaining that miserable idea. I would treat him three times a week, and he would get on his inversion table two or three times per day.

Wow, did that ever pay off! Not only did Steve fully rehabilitate his lower back, but he returned to his team the next year to win the national title.

Ever since that experience, I have been a vehement advocate of inversion therapy, and I am delighted to see a variety of such apparatuses behind many, many locker room doors.

General Physical Secret #6:
The Best Exercise on Earth

One of those fun, silly questions I sometimes ask my nerdy self is, "If I were stuck on a deserted island, what would I do to keep myself in shape?"

The answer always comes back the same – the squat.

Here's why. First, my legs would be essential to my survival, so I'd want to make sure they were in top form. If I also put some weight on my shoulders while I did my squats and used my arms to stabilize the weight, I'd be using all my major joints and muscles, while conditioning my major body parts. By stimulating several body parts, I'd also be oxygenating all these areas, which would ensure my cardiovascular conditioning. Furthermore, the demanding nature of the squat would also require that I refine my poise and steadiness, which would help my proprioceptive facilitation (balance). (I'll talk more about this in chapter 9.)

Sometimes, just for more nerdy fun, I ask the same question to other athletes. Often, the answer comes back the same as mine—until I asked Rick Slate, the head strength and conditioning coordinator for the New York Mets. Rick bucked my system in a flash by claiming that multidirectional lunging, like a swordsmen going in for the kill, is *the bomb* for athletic conditioning.

I tried it. I thought I'd never get out of bed the next day! If you are not ready for it, you will need a wheelchair while you recuperate from the soreness. And if you do them as efficiently as Rick did, you can significantly increase your overall physical conditioning.

So, my new position is: *lunge*, baby, *lunge*!

Here's how: Lunge forward, then to the side, and then backward.

Holding a 20-pound dumbbell (or a few coconuts, if you're on my deserted island) while lunging will add to the intensity of your workout and condition your body like nothing else. Because you're lunging multidirectionally, you gain explosive power and conditioning that almost all sports require, since you may never know where your legs may have to take you next (think basketball, tennis, soccer, football). This kind of conditioning makes traditional training with a leg extension or leg curl machine obsolete since those are simply single-plane, unidirectional exercises.

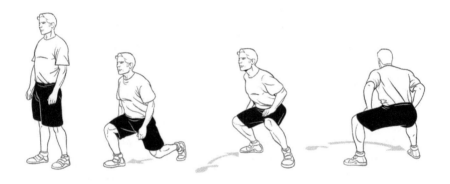

It's all pretty simple stuff. One movement, with resistance, multiple angles, it's what we do in life. Nothing we do is 100% linear. There's always a change of direction, a bump, a turn, a twist, a rotation. If life were linear, man—that would be truly boring.

Coach Rick Slate,
Strength and conditioning, New York Mets

General Physical Secret #7:
The Big O!

Here's another question I enjoy asking (myself). This may be, in part, because I'm currently an undersexed intellectual and, in part, because I know it's the question lurking beneath so many athletes' cool exteriors. Should you "shag" (bone, bang, bonk, screw, fornicate, whatever!) before a major competition?

There are two competing schools of thought on this one. *Sex School of Thought #1*: Absolutely not! Having sex before a big event will detract from the hard, aggressive behavior you need to marshal before successful competition.

Sex School of Thought #2: Absolutely yes! It calms the body and the mind, relieves stress and anxiety, and helps you focus and concentrate when the time comes.

So, in the end, the answer is … it's up to you.

There are several things to consider prior to "getting some." Will it drain you of vital neurochemicals and other hormones you need to help you maintain the intensity while competing? Could it injure your back, cause a headache, cure a headache, allow you to sleep better? Can you "play and go" or is there a lot of time-consuming romance involved? There are probably more things to consider, but you get the idea. Sex is a significant event for your body. It might be great to relax you the night before, but it may be a big drain on your body hours before a big competition.

Some athletes don't have any sex for a week or more before a big game. They believe it generates a buildup of testosterone-fueled aggression that helps pummel the opposition. On the other hand, if chess is your game, you may want to "throw down" to enhance your cerebral focus. Trusting your own body and instincts to identify what works best for you is the best approach; the right answer truly lies within you.

General Physical Secret #8:
Get Down and Dirty!

I will never, ever forget the shock of seeing what I am about to share with you.

Happily bouncing into the training room at 11:00 a.m. one recent Friday morning, I went around the corner and saw the chronically sprained ankle of an injured player being carefully treated. This player, who happened to be African American, had a history of persistent ankle swelling from even the most benign activity. At that moment, one of the athletic trainers was removing a white bandage from the player's lower leg, and I saw what appeared to be huge chunks of brown skin falling from his body. What the ...?!

I was completely aghast, as more chunks and pieces crumbled off and landed in the wastebasket below.

Huh? They were *prepared* for this abomination?

I suddenly realized that no one seemed afraid or upset. It was just another day. Upon closer examination, after refocusing my awful vision, I realized the player's ankle was encased in a thick layer of medicated clay that happened to match the color of his skin. Whew! After checking in, I was told that since this player's ankle had been such a problem, they had decided to wrap a "poultice" around it the night before to draw out the swelling.

A poultice is a concoction made from a base of special sand, dirt, or soil with a mix of herbs and other medications that are then wrapped around the injured body part. Poultices are good for stubborn strains and sprains, as well as to treat wounds where a buildup of pus needs to be drawn out. Historically, these poultices were originally used on workhorses to relieve inflammation. Ironically, I tend to see a lot of treatments invented by veterinarians that later end up "behind the locker room doors." Even more ironically, they are typically a lot cheaper when purchased from veterinarian suppliers, until they become so popular that mainstream medicine or big business figures out they can earn a hefty profit from marketing the same remedy and charging five and ten times as much for the same thing.

I'll share a good poultice mix for you to try the next time you have a bruise, strain, or sprain, which NFL superstar running back Ricky Williams, who is one of the hardest-working, mentally intense athletes I've ever seen during my career, generously gave to me. I've often heard his athletic trainers lament, "We wish we had one hundred Ricky Williamses!" Ricky's approach to wellness includes rigorous attention to his physical, mental, and nutritional needs, just as I have been suggesting throughout this book. To my great fortune, Ricky bestowed upon me one of his "secret" poultice recipes, which I am going to pass on to you:

Boil up some barbary wolfberry fruit (herb), cayenne pepper, sesame oil, and arnica to make almost a tea out of it. Then, consider one of two approaches. Either take a wash cloth, soak it in the brew, and wrap it around the injured part (consider wrapping a dry towel around the outside of the wrap to insulate and keep from making a mess). Or, make a paste out of the brew with what my mom used to use, red rock clay, similar to what you see around a baseball diamond. Then, apply a thick coat of paste around the injured area and wrap it up in a cloth bandage. Leave it on overnight and then repeat the process.

Ricky Williams,
Miami Dolphins running back,
National Football League

General Physical Secret #9:
The Electric Slide

In 1985, Dr. Robert O. Becker published his incredible book, The Body Electric.[27] In this volume, Dr. Becker discussed the principles of "Wolf's law," which describes how adaptable human tissue is (in this case, bone) when placed under certain stimulus or pressure. Providing the right amount of force or stimulus to a certain area can restructure bone. This is what occurs when the teeth are rearranged in your mouth after braces are installed or a broken bone is corrected.

Dr. Becker identified that, when a salamander grows a new tail, it is actually creating a regenerative environment for its body to heal and develop new tissue. By studying how salamanders do this, he realized that human bones could also regenerate themselves faster using a slight electrical charge. Again, we borrow from veterinary science by looking at treatment for racehorses. Instead of taking horses with fractured bones out to pasture and "euthanizing" them, or sending them to the glue factory, veterinarians discovered that they could drill holes on either side or end of the fracture site and place very low amplitude,

---

27   Becker, Robert, *The Body Electric*. (New York: William Morrow Company, Inc, 1985).

electrically charged rods into the holes to help heal the fracture. At the very least, it preserves the horse's life; at best, it may enable the horse to continue competing.

Somewhere, some smart athletic doctor figured out that what's good for the four-legged creatures must also be good for the two-legged variety. As such, it's now pretty standard practice that when a player sustains a fracture along a certain bone, portholes are drilled into the cast, and then steel rods are dropped in and laid on opposite ends of the fracture site. This creates an electrical "force field" for optimal healing (please pardon my sounding like Captain Kirk from *Star Trek* here).

Today, there's no longer any need to drill portholes in the cast or even place electrically charged metal posts into the injured site. Now, doctors use a lightweight apparatus that latches around the whole cast, and clinical studies have shown an increased site healing while simultaneously encouraging the body's own healing process with only 30 minutes of stimulation per day.[28] The average doctor would be unlikely to tell you or even know about this.

General Physical Secret #10:
Too Hot to Handle

Back in the day, the only heat rub we had was Ben-Gay. Now, innumerable products have jumped on the muscle-soothing bandwagon,

---

28   D. Beigler, et al., "Multicenter Nonunion Clinical Investigation of the CMF OL1000 Bone Growth Stimulator," *White Paper*, 1994, [PDF - 4MB]; Linovitz, et al. "Combined Magnetic Fields Accelerate and Increase Spine Fusion: A Double-Blind, Randomized, Placebo Controlled Study," *Spine* 27:13 (2002): 1383-88, [available online]; J. A. Longo, "Successful Treatment of Recalcitrant Nonunions With Combined Magnetic Field Stimulation," *Ortho Surg (Surgical Technology International VI)* (2000): 397–403, CMF OL1000 Post-Registry Data, [PDF]; J. T. Ryaby JT, et al. "The Role of Insulin-like Growth Factor II in Magnetic Field Regulation of Bone Formation," *Bioelectrochemistry and Bioenergetics* 35 (1994): 87–91; R. J. Fitzsimmons, J. T. Ryaby, et al. "Combined Magnetic Fields Increase IGF-II in TE-85 Human Osteosarcoma Bone Cell Cultures," *Endocrinology* 136 (1995): 3100–06; K. J. McLeod and C. T. Rubin, "The Effect of Low-Frequency Electrical Fields on Osteogenesis," *The Journal of Bone and Joint Surgery* 74-A,6 (1992):920–29, [available online].

each claiming they are the best formula for quick and efficient healing. Here's what I know. There is only one formula used in just about every locker room or athletic trainer's bag across the country: Cramergesic.

I developed a healthy respect for National Hockey League players while working with David Boyer, the former head athletic trainer of the Florida Panthers. One night before a game, I watched a player sidle up to David, lift his shirt, drop his pants, and silently flash his bare back and entire rear end. Without missing a beat in our conversation, David cheerfully donned a rubber glove. Fearfully envisioning a very unpleasant prostate exam, I could no longer concentrate on a word David was saying. Then, adding to my alarm, he picked up a jar of the hottest Cramergesic liniment, and I felt my knees go limp.

Four gloved fingers scooped out a gob of ointment.

He began to ...

Oh, thank Heaven!

Rub it on the athlete's entire back and upper buttocks!

After giddily realizing there would be no red-hot rectal exam, I began wondering about the wisdom of using an extremely hot liniment on such a large body surface. To the best of my knowledge, this stuff was supposed to be used on small, focal-point areas due to the intensity of its heat. After David finished shellacking the player's entire back and upper buttocks, the grateful player pulled up his pants, dropped his shirt, and silently walked away.

Stunned by this well-choreographed interaction, I timidly asked, "Umm, David, I know you are a sharp guy, and far be it from me to question your treatment protocols, but don't you think you should have wiped off some of that stuff?"

He responded with his usual seriousness, "Nah, he likes it that way."

"But Dave," I responded, "c'mon, he's gonna sweat, and that stuff is going to drip down the crack of his butt and all the sensitive membranes around his ... you know."

Dave interrupted with a chuckle and said, "Oh, don't worry, I've been through this with him before—he just says it helps him play harder!"

Even though these products were never meant to be used this way, the whole concept on which they are based is called the principle of "counter-irritation." It's the same neurological principle that explains why a scratch feels so good to an itch; you override the subtle stimulation of the itch with a massive, overwhelming, sharp-nailed scratch. In the case of sore muscles, the heat from an ointment essentially overwhelms the soreness of that muscle, while the heat brings blood flow to the affected area. This effectively "washes out" the body's natural chemical byproducts, which result in soreness from a hard workout—in other words, what you have probably heard referred to as "lactic acid buildup."

Heating ointments have been around a long time and are good when used properly, such as before an activity when your muscles are sore. However, if your pain persists beyond the ability of the heating ointment to heal, you could be covering up something much worse. So be careful if you experience the same pain and soreness for more than three to four days.

General Physical Secret #11:
The Hyperbaric Chamber

When I was growing up, I recall hearing that the only hyperbaric chamber for thousands of miles around was in the Florida Keys because it was a haven for deep-sea divers. An entire room was dedicated to this big, steel decompression tank similar to that of early MRI or CT scanners. I later learned that hyperbaric chambers actually began as far back as the mid 1600s, but were not used safely until the 1930s to help treat divers with decompression sickness.[29] Even though a couple of conditions, such as certain bacterial infections (gangrene) and carbon monoxide poisoning, had historically been treated with hyperbaric oxygen, it wasn't until about twenty years ago that hyperbaric therapy started being used to accelerate the resolution of open wounds.[30] Specifically, it was used for treatment

---

29   G. Haux, *History of Hyperbaric Chambers*, (Flagstaff, Arizona: Best Publishing, 2000).

30   W. H. Brummelkamp, Hogendijk J, Boerema I, "Treatment of anaerobic infections (clostridial myositis) by drenching tissues with oxygen under high atmospheric pressure," *Surgery* 49 (10610): 299; G. Smith and G. R. Sharp, "Treatment of coal gas poisoning with oxygen at two atmospheres pressure," *Lancet* 1 (1962): 816.

among amputees and diabetic patients with chronic, festering wounds that did not respond to conventional therapy. Hyperbaric therapy forces oxygen to circulate into distal regions of the extremities, thus facilitating the healing process.

Michael Jackson took a lot of heat for buying one of these chambers for personal health and longevity. In retrospect, he was slightly ahead of his time, as we now see, some fifteen years later, several pro athletes who have purchased portable, home-use machines to enhance and speed their recovery processes. Moreover, there has recently been some interesting research on the effectiveness of hyperbaric oxygen therapy on children with cerebral palsy and autism.[31] While probably not the easiest and most available strategy for the everyday athlete like you and me, hyperbaric oxygen therapy is worth knowing about in the context of what the superstars are doing to heal themselves.

General Physical Secret #12: Up and At 'Em

When an indifferent doctor tells you to rest in bed and then to take these drugs or those, you may want to consider getting a second opinion. If your doctor spent a whole three minutes with you or indeed never even examined you before diagnosing your ailment and calling in his prescription, that's not health care! At best, it's pain and symptom care, and at worst, it's neglect. While it might eliminate your pain in the short run, for the long haul, it's often a setup for very unpleasant long-term consequences.

31 J. P. Collet, M. Vanasse, P. Marois, M. Amar, J. Goldberg., J. Lambert, et al. "Hyperbaric oxygen for children with cerebral palsy: A randomized multicentre trial," *The Lancet* (2001) 357, 582–586; D. Montgomery, J. Goldberg, M. Amar, V. Lacroix, J. Lecomte, J. Lambert, M. Vanasse, and P. Marois, "Effects of hyperbaric oxygen therapy on children with spastic diplegic cerebral palsy: A pilot project," *Undersea and Hyperbaric Medicine* 26(4) (1999) 235–242.; D. J. Russell, P. L. Rosenbaum, D. T. Cadman, C. Gowland, S. Hardy,, and S. Jarvis, "The gross motor function measure: A means to evaluate the effects of physical therapy," *Developmental Medicine & Child Neurology* 31(3) (1989), 341–352; D. A. Rossignol, "Hyperbaric oxygen therapy might improve certain pathophysiological findings in autism," *Medical Hypotheses* 68 (6) (2007): 1208–27.

When an athlete fractures a bone, he or she starts activity again *within days* of being casted. Prolonged muscular inactivity inevitably leads to a loss of muscle mass and functional capacity (for example, strength, stamina, and coordination), which is a recipe for athletic disaster. Within two to three days of a an athlete having a fracture casted or following surgery, the athletic trainers and physical therapists will drop electrodes down the cast and to start a flurry of muscular contractions to keep atrophy at bay.

Here is what the superstar athletes' health-care providers know about the dangers of "bed rest" that your average, well-intentioned doctor doesn't:

- Degeneration of muscle fibers (atrophy) occurs within 8-10 days.
- Protein in muscle fibers begins to degrade when weight-bearing forces are considerably reduced or eliminated.
- Your body's ability to absorb oxygen decreases by 25 percent after 20 consecutive days of bed rest.
- Prolonged physical inactivity decreases the amount of blood that is pumped out of the heart (cardiac output).
- Aerobic capacity decreases by an average of 1 percent for each day of inactivity.
- Bed rest leads to an overall loss of aerobic capacity and stamina.
- You must use resistance exercise in order to prevent muscle strength deterioration.[32]

Continuing to do some controlled exercise introduces a series of stresses that cause the body to adapt, both structurally or functionally, to the physical stress. Ultimately, such activity enables the body to respond increasingly better to subsequent pressure. By the time the patient (athlete) is ready for full activity, he or she has less risk of reinjury or compensatory injury (injury to another body part), and decreased downtime due to the accelerated adaptability of the injured tissues. In other words, your body will continuously adapt to slowly increasing pressure. Too much pressure will cause it to fall apart

32   B. Saltin and L. B. Rowell, "Functional adaptations to physical activity and inactivity," *Federation Proceedings* 39 (1980): 1506–1510; J. E. Greenleaf "Intensive exercise training during bed rest attenuates deconditioning," *Medicine and Science in Sports and Exercise* 29 (1997): 207–215.

(reinjure), and insufficient pressure will result in slow, and potentially, impaired healing.

In addition to its benefits for healing your injury, aerobic exercise (for example, a treadmill or elliptical machine) and weight training have been shown to have positive effects in other important functional areas, such as glucose tolerance, insulin sensitivity, bone density, energy metabolism, and mental stability. More importantly, exercise may be one of the most effective and least costly interventions that you can performed at home. And the equipment required (handheld weights, such as dumbbells) is inexpensive.

This is a great strategy unless, of course, you want "bed rest and TV," in which case I suggest you blow off everything I just said and go on a cruise.

General Physical Secret #13:
The Pink Pad

Quite possibly, one of my favorite "secrets" is "the pink pad," or Polymem, for wound healing because it is responsible for one of the most remarkable demonstrations of healing I've ever seen. Moreover, it is a great example of how treatments in one sport (for example, baseball) can easily crossover to another (for example, football) simply as a result of who knows whom.

Here's what happened. Larry Star, the head athletic trainer for the 1997 World Series-winning Florida Marlins, made an enthusiastic call to Kevin O'Neil, the head athletic trainer for the Miami Dolphins. He talked excitedly about a pink bandage that could heal open wounds faster than anything he'd ever seen. He described how one of his baseball players had a fresh abrasion the length of his forearm. Star had heard about this cute little piece of pink material that might eliminate this nasty wound somewhat faster than conventional bandages could. However, he only had a piece long enough to cover about half of the abrasion, so he decided to put it only on the worst part of the wound. After a few days, he was astonished to discover that the worst portion of the injury had healed faster and better than the conventionally covered and less badly injured side, and hence, his enthusiastic call to Kevin. Ever since then, the "pink pad," branded as Polymem, is increasingly becoming standard practice in various athletic locker rooms across the country.

I now use it on my children whenever they'll let me. They are still young and are very seduced by the fancy and colorful characters marketed by popular commercial brands. Not to mention, what boy child, who is busy developing his strong, masculine ego, wants to walk around with a "little pink pad" on his arm?

General Physical Secret #14:
Those Irritating Bumps and Bruises

If you want to see an amazingly fast resolution of a bruise on a child, try using a homeopathic remedy that includes belladonna, arnica, chamomilla, and several other herbs. I don't see this used in too many training facilities, but my own experience is that using the cream on myself or my children has been fascinating. The best brand is probably Traumeel, and I keep a tube handy at all times, ready to slather it on when my boys get banged up. The key is to put it on right away so the anti-inflammatory effects quickly dissipate the potential bruising. It is also a helpful alternative for kids who hate using ice following an injury, like mine do.

Summary

The most important thing for you to remember from this chapter is that your body is a very slick machine composed of some very intricate and interdependent parts. In this chapter, I have given you 13 great secrets used by top athletes and their support staff to effectively manage overall physical health resulting from injury.

Here's a recap of my Ultimate Physical Strategies for Overall Body Healing, Strength, and Conditioning:

General Physical Secret #1: Going Hot and Cold ... Not Fickle, Just Sensible! After an injury, use only ice for the first 72 hours. You are free to use heat after that.

General Physical Secret #2: Don't Just Ice It—RICE It! Following an injury, use the RICE system: Rest, Ice, Compression, and Elevation.

General Physical Secret #3: S-T-R-E-T-C-H It Out. For increased muscle length and flexibility, use *moist* heat, then stretch the muscle, then massage. Repeat the process, using gradually increasing pressure on the muscle, and you'll see great results over time.

General Physical Secret #4: Rubber—It's Not Just for Tires Anymore. Rubber tubing is among the most versatile, inexpensive, and flexible accessories for enhancing your exercise routine.

General Physical Secret #5: Conversion to Inversion. An inversion table reverses the natural downward pull of gravity and gives your overused spine and hip joints a break.

General Physical Secret #6: The Best Exercise on Earth. It's simple but not easy—multidirectional lunges are the bomb for overall strength and conditioning.

General Physical Secret #7: The Big O! Sex—have it or don't; it's completely up to you. Just remember to pay attention to your own body and what it lets you know its needs are.

General Physical Secret #8: Get Down and Dirty! Dirt and mud poultices provide some of the best overall healing for wounds and bruises.

General Physical Secret #9: The Electric Slide. Using a small, electric charge stimulates injured muscles and prevents atrophy from lack of use and stimulation.

General Physical Secret #10: Too Hot to Handle. One word: Cramergesic.

General Physical Secret #11: The Hyperbaric Chamber. Hyperbaric therapy forces oxygen to circulate into distal regions of the extremities, thus facilitating the healing process.

General Physical Secret #12: Up and At 'Em. No rest for the weary; after an injury, get up and moving as fast as you can to minimize weak muscles, avoid reinjury or compensatory injury, and bring healing blood flow to the injured area.

General Physical Secret #13: The Pink Pad. The Polymem pad—the best little pad around for rapid and effective wound healing.

General Physical Secret #14: Those Irritating Bumps and Bruises. Use homeopathic Traumeel made of belladonna, arnica, chamomilla, and several other herbs to help resolve everyday bumps and bruises.

Like the secrets I offered in the other chapters, these are useful to keep around, as you may need a quick and handy reference to deal with some ailment. And, like all my other secrets, these too are available to you, already typed and organized for your convenience, at www. DrSpencerBaron.com.

Some of you may have already noticed that what's missing from this chapter are specific remedies for specific ailments to specific parts of your body—your aching feet, your sore back, your hamstrung hamstrings, and more. Yup, you guessed it, stick around because chapter 9 deals with just that, and I'm pretty sure you'll find the information there relevant and useful for what ails you.

Chapter 9:

THE ESSENTIAL ATHLETE:

Ultimate Physical Strategies for *Specific Body Part* Healing, Strength, and Conditioning

I've now shared most of my secrets for creating a mentally, nutritionally, and physically powerful and athletic body. I have one more set of secrets I want to share with you to complete this holistic model for overall conditioning, maintenance, and well-being. This last set of secrets deals with specific ailments that may afflict your body and for which you may want a particular remedy. These are problems that may affect some unique body part, such as your feet, your knees, your neck, or some other area. In this chapter, I offer you some very specific strategies for remedying your aches and pains and give you ways to avoid those discomforts in the future.

Ready ... set ... let's go!

Specific Physical Secret #1:
Happy Feet

Are you preparing for a long charity walk? Or how about a trip to New York or London, where walking is an all-day event? Believe it or not, marbles and toilet tissue are just the things to get your feet in tip-top shape. You see, the bottoms of your feet use several muscles that are responsible for each and every step. Most of the time, these amazing supports go unnoticed, until a long day of walking or running leaves them sore and achy, and each step seems agonizing. However, there is an easy way to both prevent the soreness and to take care of feet that are already beat.

Got some marbles, or more likely, several sheets of toilet tissue? Just throw them down in a small group on a carpet or a towel and, while sitting, pick them up, one by one, with your toes and then move each one to another spot about a foot or two away. To strengthen the muscles, use your toes to bunch up the toilet tissue into little balls. In addition, you can gently put pressure on a few marbles and roll them across the bottom of your feet, which will knead (or massage) the muscles at the same time. This is another way to loosen the muscles or train the feet with some definite encouragement.

For many of you, it may be best to start by using a tennis ball to begin loosening the muscles at the bottom of your feet, but if you're feeling tough, use a golf ball instead. To prepare for a race or walk, start doing this several weeks in advance so you can condition your feet to some different types of stimulus.

Orthotics

While we're on the subject of happy feet, one of the coolest comments anyone ever shared with me notes how important the right foot-wear is. "Once your foot hits the ground, anything could go wrong if there is a poor foundation." Don't stint on your shoes; proper footwear can truly make you or break you.

But not all shoes are created equally, and no two sets of feet are identical either. We each have a unique footprint, and a custom-made orthotic should not be something done only on rare occasion or because there is something "wrong" with your feet. While most of us can get away with a generically made shoe, there are so many variations in a foot that can affect your athletic performance (as well as your comfort and well-being during most any activity) if you don't care for your feet properly.

One of the most common, but typically overlooked, causes of discomfort is when one leg is longer than the other. This problem can be corrected with a small heel lift; the orthotic will naturally conform to the irregular surfaces of the feet and provide stability and support where needed. Be cautious, however; there are only a small percentage of health-care providers who can properly determine a true leg-length deficiency (as indicated by your skeleton). While a podiatrist cannot diagnose this problem, he or she can give you a good custom-made orthotic to adjust for foot problems and other abnormalities.

The best way to identify "long leg syndrome" is through an X-ray of the pelvis while standing in a weight-bearing position. Oftentimes, an aggravated stress fracture may be the cause of the longer leg. This can be easily corrected to get you back into action.[33] To alleviate some discomfort, you could start with a simple orthotic available over the counter at your local pharmacy and see if that eases some of your soreness over the first week or two. The first time you try it, you may want to wear your orthotic for only a few hours a day; then you can gradually increase your usage until you are used to wearing the orthotic full time, and then you can run in it. Your health-care professional can suggest your next step; a custom-made orthotic can range from $100 to $350 for a pair. If your doctor says it will cost any more than that, be sure to ask him if you'll also be able to walk on water while wearing it!

So how do the record-breaking distance-running Kenyan athletes run barefoot? Because they have adapted to their environment over many generations. Similarly, we have adapted to the comfort of wearing shoes and, thus, have developed particular sensitivities that make us prone to a different set of injuries than our barefoot brethren on the other side of the planet.

---

33   K. G. Bennell, Matheson, and W. Meeuwisse , "Risk factors for stress fractures," *Sports Medicine* 28(2) (1999): 91–122.

Morning Foot and Heel Pain

One morning, at the crack of dawn, I had just seen one of my former professional athlete patients, and he was walking like a frail old lady who just had a hip replacement. Somehow, despite his strange gait, he seemed to be in excellent shape.

"Why in the world are you walking like that?" I asked.

I'd heard the response before from runners; every morning he awoke with sensational heel and sole pain when he got out of bed and stepped down onto the floor. I asked him a series of questions:

"Does it ease off by the later part of the morning?"

"Yes," he answered.

"Does it feel better when you walk on the carpet versus the bare floor?"

"Yes."

"Have you been running a lot or have you slightly increased the distance or frequency of your run?"

"Yes."

"Do you sleep on your belly or on your back?"

"Belly."

"If I put my finger on your heel or arch of the foot, does it hurt?"

"Yeah, big time."

"Does aspirin or medication help?"

"For a day or two; then it comes back with a vengeance."

He asked if I thought he had a heel spur, but I said that it didn't really matter. We've X-rayed people with this kind of foot pain, and there is not a significant correlation with whether or not they have a heel spur.

In desperation, he asked, "What do I do?!"

"Simple! Get a plantar fascia night splint."

"A what??"

"A plantar fascia night splint."

Here's what was causing his pain (and maybe yours, too) and how this splint can help. The muscles that attach from your heel to your toes and are responsible for your arch have been so strained and irritated during the day that, when you go to sleep, they just want to heal. However, it's particularly painful when you sleep on your stomach; these muscles have a harder time healing when they're in the shortened state caused by that position (picture your foot flat versus when your toe is pointed as it would be when lying on your stomach. Get the idea?). When you rise in the morning, your feet stretch into a flat position, which tears the scar tissue that was busy forming overnight. Think of it this way: Remember how, when you scraped your knee or elbow, it eventually formed a scab to help it heal? And remember how, every time you bent your joint, that scab would open up and bleed because the scar was not yet flexible tissue? This is the same idea—it just happens inside, rather than outside, your body.

The night splint will hold the muscles in a stretched position overnight so they can heal properly and, by morning, you will be ready to dance—depending, of course, on how badly they've been aggravated. In general, the sooner you handle this, the better.

The Wonders of Foam Rubber

A small, square piece of foam can facilitate essential neurological healing for an injured athlete's foot or ankle or knees or hips—basically any lower extremity. It is also a great way to enhance a developing child's sense of balance, as well as mediate the effects of diminishing coordination in an elderly person. What can we learn from this? What I am going to tell you is as essential for the toddler just starting to walk and learning to master balance as for the elderly person trying to regain shaky balance so he or she doesn't fall and fracture fragile bones. Listen up, because I am about to present "Neurology 101 for Feet." And I'm going to make it ridiculously simple—"Neurology 101 for Feet for Dummies" (not that you're a dummy, of course).

Ready?

The average person has four basic nerve types: nerves that allow you to feel pain, nerves that allow you to feel just pressure, nerves that allow you to feel temperature (hot and cold), and, finally, some very neglected nerves for proprioception.

Pro ... prio ... *what*?

/Pro-prio-sep-shun/. These nerves are critical to athletic, pediatric development and recovery. These nerves allow you to run up steps without looking down to make sure you don't trip. These nerves allow a professional soccer player to look somewhere other than his feet when kicking toward the goal or a wide receiver to catch a football while his eyes are scanning for who may be about to tackle him. Providing strength and stability to the developing, aging, or injured joint is the key to reducing the potential for injury.

Here are some progressively more difficult exercises for the lower extremities that can be done with a commercially available foam balance pad. If you purchase a pad, it should be one that measures 16½" x 19½" x 2½" thick.

- One-leg balance: Try to stand on one leg for 10-30 seconds.
- One-leg balance with eyes closed: Stand on one leg for as long as possible with your eyes closed.
- Balance pad ball toss: While balancing on a balance pad, catch and toss a small (5 pound) medicine ball with a partner.
- Balance pad with half squats: While balancing on a balance pad, perform ten slow, controlled half squats.
- Step up onto balance pad: Place a balance pad six to eight inches higher than the floor, (use a small stool, step, or device to raise your step). Step up ten times.
- Step down onto balance pad: Place a balance pad six to eight inches lower than your starting point. Step down ten times.
- Lateral plyometrics: Perform a lateral (sideways) step down and then step up.

Add the exercises slowly over several weeks as tolerated. You may want to consider working with your own sports-oriented chiropractor, athletic trainer, or physical therapist to design the best program for your specific needs.

There are so many more examples, as this is a critical regimen that is very often integrated into the treatment regimen prescribed for any recovering athlete. For additional strengthening exercise with foam, you can go online and see what you find under "foam therapy balance pads" or "balance blocks."

Specific Physical Secret #2:
Get Your Head on Straight, Please!

This is all about getting your head screwed on straight.

Did you know that all the nerves from your brain and spinal cord control pretty much your whole body? That said, it should be no surprise that the nerves that branch off the neck and run through the upper region of the spinal bones are responsible for sending and receiving critical impulses from all the upper extremities, and these are vitally important to *all* sports that require upper body strength, stamina, and dexterity. These are also extremely important in maintaining balance, or proprioception, as we just discussed above.

Most of you use your arms for both your work and your play. Arms are pretty important to just about all aspects of your day-to-day functioning (imagine trying to take a shower or eat breakfast or even locate and change the channel on the TV remote control without your arms). If you are just fine with merely being able to plant both feet on the ground after the alarm clock goes off, then you have my full permission to just ...

Stop reading this book.

But if you want more, then read on.

You can improve your coordination and reflexes by having the neck bones adjusted or manipulated. There are several reasons you should want to do this. First, being successful at most sports requires excellent coordination. Second, fast and agile reflexes are what make a good athlete great; it's pretty hard to be a superior player if your reflexes or coordination are off. Third, and perhaps most important to the average person, sudden or increasing lack of coordination can be a sign of more serious problems. That is, if you start to notice that your coordination is faltering, it may be a sign that the nerves that control your balance (or proprioception) are impeded, and you'll want to get that taken care of as soon as possible. Chiropractic is absolutely one of the best ways to keep the nerves that control balance and reflexes as healthy as possible.

Consider this: The next time a glass of milk teeters off the counter near your child, you may wish you had the instinctive catlike reflexes of tennis superstar Roger Federer. Among other superstar athletes, Roger has regular chiropractic adjustments to ensure that his nerves and reflexes stay in peak shape. It is increasingly becoming accepted practice for all kinds of major sports athletes to get their spines adjusted by a skilled chiropractor.

Spinal manipulation is meant to restore normal motion to aching, sore, and stiff joints. It is also designed to maximize optimal brain, spinal cord, and nerve function, which is the lifeline to every system in your whole body. In the United States, spinal manipulation is done primarily by doctors of chiropractic, and the purpose of their work is to restore normal motion to the bones of the spine (or extremities) where the "field of motion [has become] too great in some directions and too small in others."[34] This is not to suggest that the bones are "out of place," like a brick in a wall needing to be knocked back in. Rather, chiropractic physicians identify deviations from normal motion that may be due to inflammation or scar tissue and then adjust the bones in your spine to ensure that your nerves remain unrestricted and can carry essential messages to all your organs and extremities. Many painful conditions can arise from what is actually a relatively simple problem of nerves irritated by deviated spinal bones.

Specific Physical Secret #3: You're No Knucklehead!

"Don't *ever* crack your knuckles!"

Or so they say.

But who are "they"? Well, if you are anything like me, they was your mom, your mom's mom, and her mom before her. For generations, we've heard that cracking knuckles would make them big, fat, and arthritic. Well, I am happy to report that this is simply *not* true, and you have my permission to crack away as much as you like.

One report documented the experience of a man who cracked the knuckles of his left hand at least twice a day for 50 years. He left his right hand relatively untouched. Thus, he cracked the knuckles on his right hand at least 36,500 times, while he cracked those on his right hand rarely and only spontaneously. After 50 years, his hands were

---

34   R. A. Leach (ed.), "Chapter 2: History of the Chiropractic Theories," *The Chiropractic Theories: A Textbook of Scientific Research*, edition 4 (Baltimore: Lippincott, Williams & Wilkins, 2004), 19.

compared for the presence of arthritis. Lo and behold, there was no arthritis in either hand.[35]

Over the years, several athletes have requested my spinal adjusting services for their fingers and wrists. At first, I thought, why not? They continued to return with significant praise and ongoing requests for such manipulation. I wondered why this had such a "feel good" response since the joints of the spine were structurally more sophisticated that the fingers. Here is what I found:

Two studies examined what we refer to as "cracking" in human joints.[36] Both studies found that "cracking" a knuckle resulted in a gas bubble leaving the joint. One study found the gas to be "greater than 80 percent CO_2."[37] CO_2, or carbon dioxide, is the same stuff we produce when exhaling and is used by plants to survive. So, one might hypothesize that the reason it feels good is because eliminating gas from a closed space reduces the pressure within that space. Now, we all know about the undeniable pleasure of relieving gas from an enclosed space (think lower intestine here). I guess it would be polite to say, "Excuse me," when cracking your knuckles, since you are "passing gas" there, too.

Specific Physical Secret #4:
Hamstrung by Your Hamstrings

It's not big news that stretching your muscles is good practice, and stretching the hamstrings is often first on the stretching to-do list. Unfortunately, this may be among the more antiquated approaches to adequately preparing for an athletic event. In fact, many injuries can occur using traditional runners' stretches like throwing your leg onto the bumper of a nearby car and lunging into it. Although it may feel good momentarily, these repetitive short, bouncing actions

---

35   D. Unger, "Does knuckle cracking lead to arthritis of the fingers?" *Arthritis & Rheumatism* 41(5) (1998): 949–50.

36   J. B. Roston and R. Wheeler-Haines R, "Cracking in the metacarpo-phalangeal joint." *Journal of Anatomy* 81(1947):165–173; A. Unsworth, D. Dowson, and V. Wright, "'Cracking joints': A bioengineering study of cavitation in the metacarpo-phalangeal joint." *Annals of the Rheumatic Diseases* 30(4) (1971): 348–58.

37   Unsworth (1971), 350.

can easily strain the muscle and create microscopic rips and tears that may eventually cause big problems.

Current thought suggests that the best way to prepare a muscle to handle stress is not to stretch, but to *warm up*. The most effective approach is to actually *do* the activity you are about to engage in, gradually increasing degrees. So, if you are a runner, then you should walk first and then go into a very light jog, gradually increasing your speed and intensity before your full-out run. This way, you are slowly and gradually engaging the small, intrinsic muscles that you'll need for maximum performance. This is how top sprinters from all over the world get ready to compete.

Here's an approach to hamstring maintenance that I learned from my friend Ben Westby, Assistant Athletic Trainer of the Miami Dolphins. I've been doing this for over a year now, following a first-time hamstring tear that was hanging me up for months. He calls it the "90–90 wall hemi-bridge" (yeah, weird name, isn't it?), and you should do it right before your run. You should also do this several times a week to strengthen the hamstrings, which are so prone to strain on a runner. Here is how to do it:

> *Lie on your back with your knees and hips both bent at 90 degrees, with the soles of your feet flat against a wall. Do a pelvic tilt and lift your butt off the ground about an inch. Try to isolate your hamstring muscles as you do this. Hold this position with your left leg and straighten your right leg. Lower and raise your straight right leg. Keeping it straight, touch your heel on and off the wall. Breathe normally. Keep your pelvis tilted in "up" position. Do this 10 to 15 times, and then switch legs. Perform two to three sets.*

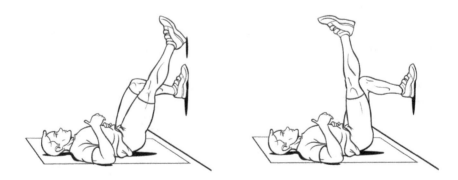

Specific Physical Secret #5:
Abs-olutely the Best

Want six-pack abs? Despite all the various claims of TV and magazine advertisements featuring sexy, chiseled abdominal muscles achieved quickly, painlessly, and inexpensively. Here's what I've learned and what the professionals actually do.

As I've mentioned, I competed as a teenage wrestler and later as an amatuer bodybuilder for many years. I won several titles ranging from first through fifth place in several events like the Mr. Florida, Mr. Southern States, and USA competitions. In order to get that far in such competitions, I had to understand how to achieve physical symmetry and to get that "ripped" look, which essentially means having the most muscle with the least body fat. As a result of these experiences, I spent a lot of time and energy searching for and finding the most effective and least injurious abdominal exercises. Trust me here; I *really* understand how muscles respond to conditioning and resistance training.

During my intensive search for the most effective and efficient muscle conditioning practices, I came across several studies touting "the best" practices for abdominal conditioning.[38] However, each one was similarly, and critically, flawed – not one of them either considered or evaluated the potential damage to the lower back. By far, the best book I've ever seen on abdominal conditioning is *The Complete Book of Abs* by Kurt and Brett Brungardt[39] and, even though it was published a decade

---

38   F. Barnett and W. Gilleard, "The use of lumbar spinal stabilization techniques during the performance of abdominal strengthening exercise variations," *Journal of Sports Medicine and Physical Fitness* 45(1) (2005): 38–43, Institute of Sport and Exercise Science, James Cook University, Townsville QLD, Australia; D. M. Urquhart, P. W. Hodges, T. J. Allen, and I. H. Story, "Abdominal muscle recruitment during a range of voluntary exercises," *Manual Therapy* 10(2):144-53; R. F. Escamilla, M. S. McTaggart, E. J. Fricklas, R. DeWitt, P. Kelleher, M. K. Taylor, A. Hreljac, and C. T. Moorman, "An electromyographic analysis of commercial and common abdominal exercises: implications for rehabilitation and training," *Journal of Orthopedic Sports Physical Therapy* 36(2) (2006): 45–57.

39   K. Brungardt and B. Brungardt, *The Complete Book of Abs*, (New York: Random House 1998).

ago in 1998, abdominal exercises have not changed. The only exercise I ever found that, to this day, remains the most scientifically sound, is the "V-Up." This exercise is still the most effective for the abdominals while having the least effect on the low back. Here's how to do it:

Lie flat on the floor. Extend your legs and arms straight up to the ceiling. Now, touch your fingers to your toes. Hold this position for five seconds. Start with 10-15 repetitions. Increase gradually as you get stronger. That's it.

Did you blink and miss it? Read it again.

Guess what? No low-back injury—ever (if you are doing it correctly).

Now, fast forward about 10 years to my early days as a practicing sports chiropractor, when I found myself treating a seemingly endless stream of lower-back injuries from a particular team. As I interviewed each player and reviewed his medical history, there seemed to be a common denominator in each player's experience—they were all doing the same, poorly considered and executed abdominal conditioning exercises. One by one, and unbeknownst to each other, each player's lower back was being similarly decimated by these damaging exercises. So, I made a few subtle but key suggestions to the players about what to do and how to best communicate this proposed change in routine to their strength and conditioning coach, and soon the problem had been resolved.

Guess what they all do now? Yup, the V-up (in addition to a few other safe abdominal exercises that are not damaging to the lower back and that also strengthen other core muscles).

By the way, here's another critical tidbit that many of you may already know, but many of you may not (or may be resisting): No matter how many repetitions of an abdominal (or any other spot target conditioning) exercise you do, it *will not* spot reduce from the target location. So, put another way, one thousand sit-ups *will not* reduce body fat from your midsection any more than twenty, thirty, or forty sit-ups (or V-Ups) combined with a good diet.[40]

Specific Physical Secret #6:
Putting Your Neck on the Line

---

40   Kostek, "Subcutaneous Fat Alterations Resulting from an Upper-Body Resistance Training Program," *APPLIED SCIENCES. Medicine & Science in Sports & Exercise* 39(7) (2007): 1177–1185.

Now that you've got your head on straight, how do you keep it that way? The simplest, safest, and most practical approach to keeping your neck muscles strong and conditioned is by using your head.

That's right; just use your head.

Strengthening your neck can prevent or minimize serious injuries resulting from unexpected events such as trips and falls, auto accidents, and even a high-velocity sneeze or coughing attack. Moreover, this will help your posture, give you relief from chronic headaches, and combat the ill effects from sitting at a computer all day. I treat auto accident victims of whiplash exactly the same way I treat rodeo bull riders. Talk about a fearless athlete; no one beats the hundreds of cowboys I treated while working for Wrangler at the rodeos. I've heard it said that an eight-second bull ride is equivalent to ten rear-end motor vehicle crashes at 10–20 miles per hour. If you could take care of your neck as well as these guys, you'd have pretty amazing head and neck strength.

Here's what you do: Lie on your bed with your head hanging off the edge. Start on your back, then bring your head up and touch your chin to your chest. Repeat ten times. Next, lie on your left side and tilt your head up as if you were trying to touch your shoulder to your ear. Then, gently lower your head back down again. Repeat ten times. Now, turn your body all the way over so you are lying on your right side and do the same side-to-side motion ten times. Lastly, lie on your belly. This is the most important since it is intricately involved with good posture and can reverse some of the hunching over you do while working at the computer all day. Your chin should come all the way down in the relaxed position and then bring the whole head up and extend the head and neck like a lizard doing a mating ritual. (OK, I threw a weird visual in there just to see if you were still paying attention. Remember, I live in South Florida—I see this a lot!) Arch your neck back as far as you comfortably can, then slowly lower the head again. Repeat ten times. Do this two to four times a week, and you will be surprised by the changes in your strength and overall comfort.

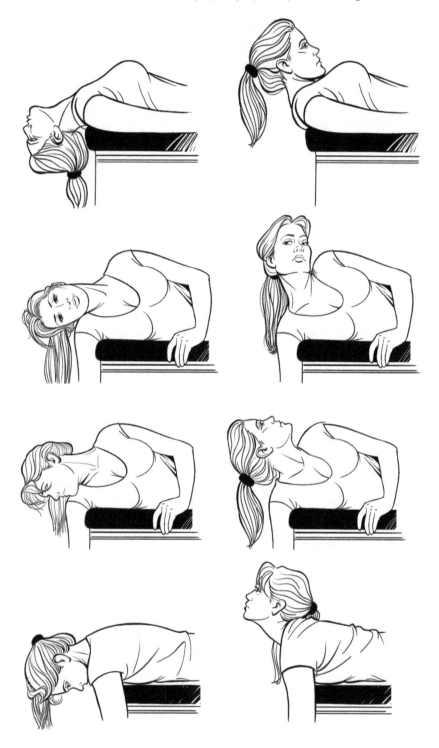

Specific Physical Secret #7:
A Sight for Sore Eyes

My vision stinks! I cannot see well during the day and, at night, it's really awful. Even with the right contacts or glasses, it doesn't matter very much. As such, I was particularly fascinated by an innovative approach to looking into the sun without sunglasses that some professional athletes shared with me. I recently found few athletes sporting these new tinted contact lenses that enabled them to look directly into the sun and still catch a ball. They really work!

The idea is to improve the athlete's ability to focus under a variety of climatologic conditions. These contact lenses come in four different varieties: golf tint, high-visibility tint, speed tint, and polarized tint. Golf tint is designed to help the golfer better distinguish the grass and the ball. High-visibility tint is designed to help the athlete see objects better in low light; it especially accentuates the color yellow. Speed tint, which works well while on the road, filters out colors that contribute to glare while putting an emphasis on the color red. Polarized tint, useful for water sports, gets rid of the glare from reflective surfaces.

You don't have to have bad vision to benefit from these lenses. However, if you are not used to wearing contact lenses, they can be distracting. The major challenge is for those who play on dirt and may have muck kicked up into their eyes. One athlete told me, "It feels like broken glass raking across your eyeball."

Specific Physical Secret #7:
Don't Go Weak at the Knees

"This is just a test. For the next sixty seconds, the Emergency Broadcast System will be conducting a test."

Remember those tedious interruptions that the Federal Communications Commission (FCC) would run in the 1970s and '80s on your TV and radio to ensure that they'd be able to warn you of impending emergencies? Well, I am not the FCC, but I am going to issue a warning about this next really cool secret.

Do you ever experience knee pain? There is one primary cause of most muscle, tendon, ligament, cartilage, vascular, lymph node, and bone problems that make your knees hurt. Here's a top secret, little-known, athlete-proven answer to most of your common, everyday knee stresses and strains that can save you lots of time and money, as well as prevent bigger knee problems later on down the road.

Ready? Here goes ...

Chondromalacia Patella, Patellofemoral Arthralgia, aka "PFA."

This complicated and unpronounceable word basically refers to pain behind the kneecap. It is often characterized by a dull ache, sometimes there might be a sharp pain with movement, especially walking up stairs or attempting to stand after sitting for a while. It may feel like a kind of grinding behind the kneecap when you put your hand over your knee and extend one leg on top of, or crossed over, the other one. Kneeling is a disaster, and running is ridiculous.

What happened here?

You have probably worn down or irritated the smooth cartilage lining behind the kneecap, which used to be there to provide that nice gliding movement while walking, jogging, or running. You may also have an imbalanced quadricep. Usually, the culprit is that one of your four primary "quad" muscles has become weak or overpowered by the other three, which has caused the tracking of your kneecap to be misaligned and thus to rub the cartilage lining more so in one area. This, in turn, has provoked overuse and irritation.

So, want to know the solution?

It's pretty simple.

You may laugh.

Duct tape. Yup, plain ole' duct tape.

Aside from taping up a broken car window, fixing a leaky pipe, and hemming your pants, all you manly men out there now have yet another use for duct tape! You can tape your knee! Be clear, this is *not* a remedy, but it is a way of testing to see if what ails you is what I am describing.

Try this: Cut yourself a three-inch long piece of duct tape. Affix one side of the tape just slightly past the outside of the tendon (see figure 11) and pull the outside over to the inside and lay down the rest of the tape at a slight angle upward. Now go try to walk

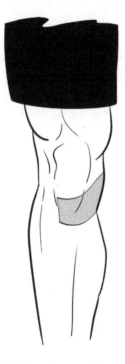

up steps or squat down. If there is no pain, you probably have the above described condition. If so, either go to your doctor and have him or her order for you, or go online and purchase, something called a "Cho-pat" or "patellar tendon knee strap." Sometimes, the changes in pain are remarkable. This is one of those real tried-and-true secrets from behind the locker room doors; athletes suffer from this all the time, and this is how they deal with it. Now, go put your duct tape to some better use, like fixing your kid's bicycle or your wife's high-heeled shoes.

Summary

The secrets I've shared with you in this section are invaluable for taking care of all the parts of your body, from the top of your head to the soles of your feet. Some of these are reactive strategies; that is, you would do them in response to a specific injury or other ailment. Many of them are preventive; you should do them all the time and thus avoid problems that may otherwise cause your body to function at less than full capacity. Here's a recap of what we covered in this chapter on "Ultimate Physical Strategies for Specific Body Part Healing, Strength, and Conditioning."

Specific Physical Secret #1: Happy Feet. Use orthotics for best shoe comfort and fit; manage morning foot and heel pain with a plantar fascia night splint; use foam rubber as an essential additive to your foot care routine.

Specific Physical Secret #2: Get Your Head on Straight, Please! Take advantage of the wonders of chiropractic medicine to keep your head and neck strong and your nervous system operating at peak capacity.

Specific Physical Secret #3: You're No Knucklehead! Cracking your knuckles will *not* give you arthritis or any other problem; crack away and enjoy it!

Specific Physical Secret #4: Hamstrung by Your Hamstrings. Be very careful how you stretch your hamstrings—use the 90–90 wall hemi-bridge for optimum strength and conditioning.

Specific Physical Secret #5: Abs-olutely the Best. Use your V-up to tone up. Don't do abdominal exercises that can hurt your back through lack of adequate support.

Specific Physical Secret #6: Putting Your Neck on the Line. Do regular neck strengthening exercises to strengthen muscles and help prevent serious injury from accidents or other unexpected events.

Specific Physical Secret #7: A Sight for Sore Eyes. Explore the possibilities of tinted contact lenses to help your eyes function best, irrespective of climatologic challenges.

Specific Physical Secret #8: Don't Go Weak at the Knees. Use duct tape to see if you have PFA, then see if a "Cho-pat" or "patellar tendon knee strap" is the right solution for your aching knees.

We've had a great run together as I've shared with you some of my best secrets for staying in peak performance condition. I'll tie it all up for you in the next chapter, and then you are on your way to the best physical, mental, and nutritional state of your whole life!

Chapter 10:

BRINGING IT ALL HOME:

Using Your New Peak Mental, Nutritional, and Physical Conditioning Strategies

Introduction

All too often, the media focuses on what is going *wrong* with professional athletes, their sports, or something else in the world of professional athletics. Headlines reading: "Wide Receiver Arrested," "Soccer Player Dies of In-Game Head Injury," or "Charges Filed Against ...," highlight the dark side of professional sports and its superstars. Sports stories are not exempt from the media mantra, "If it bleeds, it leads," and scandal, corruption, sex, and drugs are increasingly becoming more interesting than the sport itself.

There is something inherently irresponsible about such sensationalized reporting of the "news." In "The News about the News:

American Journalism in Peril"[41] Washington Post editors Leonard Downie Jr. and Robert Kaiser suggest that humans are instinctively curious. They assert that journalism relieves that curiosity, and what has passed for news in recent years has been untrustworthy, irresponsible, misleading, or incomplete. Again, sports have not been exempt from this trend.

My intention in *Secrets of the Game* has been to focus on the positive side of professional sports. My goal has been to help you uncover the secrets of how professional athletes take good care of themselves and how you can do the same. I've tried to give you insights about how athletes think, eat, care for injury, manage pain, and train their bodies and minds. My goal has been to identify what is *working* in this arena, rather than focus on what is broken.

In *Secrets of the Game*, I've brought you behind the scenes to hear some of the *good* news in professional sports. I've proffered some of the cutting-edge health-care techniques that exist to support superstar athletes so they can operate at peak performance levels for themselves, their teams, and for you, their loyal fans. But these practices no longer need to be "secrets" behind closed locker room doors. Indeed, they should be, and now increasingly are, available to each of you. You should have all the best information in order to make the best possible decisions about your own and your family's health.

Brief Review of Secrets of the Game

In chapter 1, I offered you some thoughts about how to become more responsible for your own health care and overall well-being. I suggested that you could become the architect of your own good health if you had the right information at your fingertips. I suggested that this book was one element of having such valuable information readily available.

Chapter 2 explored the history of medicine and described how it has been replete with unproven beliefs and bias. I walked you through the history of modern medicine and asserted that understanding the mind/body connection in medicine is essential to health and wellness. Homeopathy was once the standard way to treat most conditions,

---

41   L. Downie; R. Kaiser, *The News about the News: American Journalism in Peril* (Knopf: Random House, 2002), 292.

and it worked by mimicking the symptoms of an ailment, rather than covering it up with symptoms of wellness, as in current allopathic medicine. Ultimately, the best treatment uses a combination of Eastern (getting to the source of the symptoms) and Western (eliminating symptoms) practices. I proposed a new philosophy, which I called "the new mainstream," designed to integrate the best of traditional and alternative medicines as a standard and uniform approach to health care.

Finally, I advised that the easiest way to maintain health is to understand the importance of equilibrium among your mental, nutritional, and physical needs and how to keep these in healthy balance. Your greatest gift is choice, but to choose best is to be well informed.

Chapter 3 was intended to introduce you to some of the cheap and easy tricks professional athletes use to get and stay well. Treatment does not have to be expensive; it simply has to work. And many treatments are very, very affordable. Moreover, I suggested that symptoms such as pain are only a small expression of a "dis-eased" body, and that pain is the body's fire alarm. Pain is the "the tip of the iceberg," letting you know that some disorder may need more concentrated attention. I reminded you that eliminating pain does *not* convey complete health and that rather than simply masking your pain, you would be well advised to consider looking deeper to resolve the underlying problem that is causing it. "No pain, no gain" is not the healthiest approach.

In chapter 4, I asked you to consider that your mind is your most powerful tool in getting and staying healthy. I proposed the twin concepts of mental toughness and resilience as key factors in giving you a winning edge in any challenge. I also suggested that if you really want to see a winner, you should look at the losers to see how people handle losing. The ones who get defeated are the true losers, but the ones who rise to the challenge and become stronger and more resilient are the true winners, whether or not they win the game.

Concepts to help you strengthen your mind continued into chapter 5, as I asked you to consider outwitting your ineffective thinking by changing your vocabulary, resisting mind rot by avoiding negative influences, and reinforcing your thoughts by capitalizing on your own motivational masters. I told you how music can help and how to choose your music depending on your athletic goal.

Other mental tricks include monitoring your own superstitions, which have no true bearing on your ability; their power only derives from that which you give them. In addition, remember that finding heroes or finding people who exemplify the person you want to be is key and that you can leave a legacy by getting in touch with what inspires you. Remember to pay attention to your achievements, not just your defeats, and to use those small (or large) victories to continually motivate you. Remember, too, that you are competent and can accomplish anything you put your own powerful mind to. Be intentional with your thoughts, as these guide you into becoming a master of your own success.

I told you that, after learning to harness the power of your mind, it is equally important to take care of your body, and one of the most important ways to do this is through your nutrition. Chapters 6 and 7 provided basic, vital information to keep your body healthy by focusing on what you put into it. For example, monitor your water consumption with a urine color chart. Coffee is not so bad after all. Use electrolyte drinks only during and after vigorous activity; use glucosamine chondroitin to protect your joints, and cycle different foods for effective digestion. Don't forget that Mama's home recipes have a vital place in sports.

I then moved on to physical remedies to keep your body operating in peak performance shape and gave you some great tips and techniques for how to both prevent and recover from injury in chapters 8 and 9. In chapter 8, I gave you general remedies for overall body conditioning. I cleared up the when-to-use-cold-and-when-to-use-heat mystery by telling you to cool down after an injury with ice and to use heat only after the first 72 hours have passed. You can also use heat to lengthen shortened muscles. For your tired and aching feet, marbles, toilet tissue, golf balls, and tennis balls are the tools you'll need. If you want to go "high tech", use your plantar fascia night splint and orthotics in your shoes.

Moreover, in chapter 8, you learned how to affect proprioception, the neurological system for balance, by using a simple foam rubber pad and that occasionally cracking your knuckles will not increase your propensity toward arthritis. Hanging upside down may relieve joint stress and nerve pressure. Protect your hamstrings with a solid strengthening exercise and do the V-Up for abdominal conditioning. Get your neck adjusted to generate better neurological control and then strengthen the muscles for stability and protection, not to mention improving your posture. Poultices can help reduce swelling, and duct tape can help you identify what is wrong with your knees. Then there was using electricity to heal a fracture quicker and the revolutionary "pink pad" to heal a wound, fast! For the last, best exercise on Earth, try multidimensional lunges. Motion and oxygen can also improve your health and get you back in action as quickly as a multimillion-dollar professional athlete.

And then there's *sex*. Do it or don't; it's pretty much up to you.

So What's Next for You?

There are a number of ways you can use this book. On the one hand, it might make a nice doorstop or a placemat to keep your table dry. On the other hand, you could use it the way I hope you will—as a great reference book that is always available to you as a place to find good health advice. My intention is that you keep it handy for when, say, your son sprains his ankle and you wonder what to do next. (Remember— RICE it!) Or pick it up when you are struggling with how to calm your nerves and increase memory retention as you feel your mental energy slipping away. (Try slipping into something comfortable like Johann Sebastian Bach's *Largo from Harpsichord Concert in F Minor*).

You might develop your own strategies based on routine experiences in your own life or those of other people with whom you spend time. What do you do when you slam your thigh into the corner of a table and wonder how to avoid that nasty bruise you know will appear inside 24 hours—just in time for the big date and the short skirt you were hoping to wear?

Answer:

    1) Slather on some Traumeel cream or some other great source of arnica.

    2) Find a piece of "pink pad" (Polymem) and tape it to the injury before you go to sleep.

What about when your colleague has a festering blister from a new pair of "glam" shoes she insisted on wearing all day? What do you tell her?

Hey, I just read this book called Secrets of the Game *that says all the hottest sport superstars use this mix of zinc oxide and—get this—Preparation H! (You know, that stuff you use when you got a pain in the …) Go figure, but I tried it, and it really worked!"*

For more information on the "locker room remedy" for blisters, visit the website: www.DrSpencerBaron.com.

If you feel overwhelmed trying to figure out how to begin getting in shape or identifying how these strategies can help empower and support you in everyday situations, let me do the thinking for you. Here are a few combinations of mental, physical, and nutritional strategies that might work well for you (and there are many more ideas and combinations of approaches that might be just what you're looking for, on my website at www. DrSpencerBaron.com).

If you want more out of your diet, try this easy routine:

1) Drink less water during your meals.
2) Get a food sensitivity test done.
3) Start your "best abdominal exercise" (the V-Up).
4) Identify and then focus on your goal when you feel lethargic or when you have time constraints.

If you're going to ask your boss for a raise or confront your mother-in-law about her constant interference in your business or fire a poorly performing employee, try this:

1) Choose an empowered mentor whom you can model.
2) Recall time(s) you overcame great opposition.
3) Don't eat a big meal; you need all the energy and clarity you can muster.
4) Don't have sex beforehand; you may need aggressive persuasiveness.

As an athletic strategy for while you are, say, preparing for the local five-kilometer run, or the cycling club's annual long-distance ride, try this:

1) Use the strengthening maneuver for preparing your hamstrings (90–90 hemi-wall-bridge); maybe you can even smear some warming analgesic balm on your low back or calf muscles.
2) Dose up on glucosamine chondroitin to protect your joints several days ahead of time.
3) Hydrate effectively, even if it is cold out.
4) Pick some perfect music to keep you fired up and motivated.

Whatever your unique situation, there is something suitable here for you, your child, your grandparent, or just about anyone else in your life. That was how I intended the book to be used. It's not supposed to be just a ton of secrets from superstar athletes to be used by other athletes. It's for you, the "armchair athlete," the "weekend warrior," the business leader, and the trash collector. As I said in the beginning, it's all about giving you choice and power about how to create and use your own body to its best advantage, just as superstar athletes have also learned to do.

So What's Next for Me?

I sometimes wonder why I am so passionate about learning how to help people take better care of themselves. I suspect it's something about the value of a child's health, because even before I had children of my own, an appreciative hug from a child for making a painful time a little easier was about the most moving thing I could ever experience. When my first child was one year old, I got it.

Out of nowhere as I was playing with him one day, I felt tears fill my eyes. I realized that this "little man," this extraordinary gift from God, was *my* responsibility. I had to take care of him, no matter what. *No matter what.*

If you are a parent, you know what I am talking about. My commitment to continually explore better health-care choices is about ensuring that we all get the same options to be healthy, irrespective of how much money we have, who our friends are, who our parents are, what job we hold, what education we have or don't have, or any other life circumstance. We *all* deserve to be healthy. For me, *Secrets of the Game* is my first step in spreading this information far beyond the small number of people I can personally reach through individual treatment or by lecturing to groups. Hopefully, this book will reach many, many people I will never meet, and it will make a difference for them. More importantly, I hope it will make a difference for their children.

This book, and all my writing from this moment forward, is dedicated to communicating about the amazing lives that professional athletes live and what it takes to keep them strong and healthy. It's not magic; it takes years of hard work, endurance, and persistence to get where they are and stay there. You should be aware of the extremely hard work that they must master and that behind any inherent skill stands an incredibly talented and dedicated team of support staff, health-care professionals and, most of all, their families.

Athletes' health-care professionals deserve far more than the few accolades they receive. They are indeed the true contenders in the health-care arena who never stop learning what it takes to get their patients healthier, faster, and stronger each time they face the field, court, track, or stadium.

As for me, I will continue to do my part to ensure that these *secrets* become common knowledge and do not remain only behind closed locker room doors for the select few who are lucky enough to reap their benefits. The information in this book is just the beginning. I'll continue to share more in *Secrets of the Game Volume II*, as well as on the *Secrets* website (www.DrSpencerBaron.com). I will do my best to provide you continuous, up-to-date information as I lecture around the world, and I'll keep gathering new and improved data on the best, for the best, in sports health-care management. You can help by using these tools, telling your friends about them, and demanding more and better health-care options for you and your family.

In the end, if you take one great idea from this book and put it into consistent practice in your life, it may change your whole experience of your body and the amazing power it holds. This has been my life's quest, and I look forward to hearing more from you about how it's working. I'd love to hear from you with what's working and what's not and what new secrets you may have found that I should be aware of. Please email me your comments and stories to DrBaron@DrSpencerBaron.com. I can't wait to hear how *Secrets of the Game* has made a difference in your life.

My best to you,
Doc B

Oprah's Angel Network®

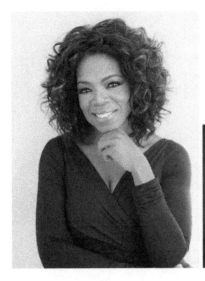 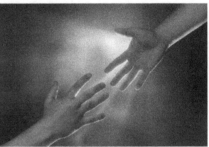

Give people the chance to live their best lives.

In an effort to support a message consistent with
Secrets of the Game,
a percentage of all book sales will go to
Oprah's Angel Network.
Get involved today, visit
www.oprahsangelnetwork.org